The Bible Promises of Healing
Vol II

Table of Contents

Introduction

Before you read this book, I highly recommend reading my first book on this topic, entitled "The Bible Promises of Healing, 16 Letters for Mom." It is available on Amazon and Audible and at these links https://rebrand.ly/Ivan-Thompson-Amazon https://rebrand.ly/Ivan-Thompson-Audible.

In this sequel, I will focus on things I did not include in the first book or only lightly touched upon. You may wonder why I didn't include the things in this book in that book. The reason is simple. I believe I have a greater revelation of the Scriptures than I had then. Further, the Bible has so much to say on the subject of healing that it is hard to capture all in one book. God's promises and His will for our healing are so extensive that it is hard to include all the places in Scripture where He shares them.

The first part of Jhn 16:13 says, "Howbeit when he, the Spirit of truth, is come, he will guide you into all truth..." Jhn 14:26 (NIV) says, "But the Advocate, the Holy Spirit, whom the Father will send in my name, will teach you all things and will remind you of everything I have said to you." When I say I have a greater revelation of the Scriptures on healing, I am referring directly to the work and ministry of the Holy Spirit. The Holy Spirit has been guiding me "into all truth" by reminding me of the things that Jesus said and is teaching me about healing by walking me through the Scriptures.

Author's Prayer

I am including the prayer that I pray as I write. My hope is that the reader would agree with the words of this prayer and get everything that God intended for them out of this book. There may be beneficial things, revelations, and clarification that God leads the reader to that aren't even written in this book.

If, as you read, the Holy Spirit leads you to other Scriptures, follow His leading. It may also be helpful to journal what the Holy Spirit brings up in your heart. Take note of things you don't understand or disagree with, and take time in prayer in communion with the Holy Spirit to carefully address them.

MY PRAYER

To be a better author, I pray that what I write will:

- Loose the light of the glorious gospel of Christ to men and women who have been blinded **2 Cor 4:4** *"In whom the god of this world hath blinded the minds of them which believe not, lest the light of the glorious gospel of Christ, who is the image of God, should shine unto them."*
- Arm God's flock

- Open the spiritual eyes, the understanding of the reader: **Eph 1:18** (NIV) *"I pray that the <u>eyes</u> of your heart may be <u>enlightened</u> in order that you may know the hope to which he has called you, the riches of his glorious inheritance in his holy people"* (KJV) "the eyes of your <u>understanding being enlightened</u>; that you may know what is the hope of His calling, what are the riches of the glory of His inheritance in the saints."
- Overcome the spirit of error: **1 Jhn 4:6 (KJV)** *"We are of God: he that knoweth God heareth us; he that is not of God heareth not us. Hereby know we the spirit of truth, and the spirit of error."*
- Result in breakthrough over religious traditions that make the Word of God of no effect in their lives: **Mark 7:13** (NKJV) *"...making the word of God of no effect through your tradition which you have handed down. And many such things you do."*
- Stir up the reader's desire to study the Word of God: **2 Timothy 2:15** *"Study to shew thyself approved unto God, a workman that needeth not to be ashamed, rightly dividing the word of truth."*
- Be shared with such simplicity and clarity that it would accomplish God's will and pierce even to the soul and spirit, i.e<u>., be impactful</u> at spirit,

soul, and heart level and have the ability to discern/correct thoughts and intents of the heart or will: **Hebrews 4:12** *"For the word of God is quick, and powerful, and sharper than any two-edged sword, piercing even to the dividing asunder of soul and spirit, and of the joints and marrow, and is a discerner of the thoughts and intents of the heart."*

- That the Spirit of the Lord would be upon me (**Isa 61:1, Luke 4:18**) as I write so that through me yokes would be destroyed, liberty would be proclaimed to the captives/bruised, prison doors would be opened, heaviness would be lifted, the brokenhearted would be healed, deliverance would be preached, the blind would recover their sight and see the light of the glorious gospel of Christ, the "good news" found in the entirety of the gospel (that they prosper and be in health, spirit soul and body (**3 Jhn 1:2**)

The Importance of Hearing

"So then faith comes by hearing, and hearing by the word of God."

Rom 10:17 (NKJV)

"Therefore we ought to give even more earnest heed to the things which we have heard, lest at any time we should let them slip."

Heb 2:1

"Yet the news about him spread all the more, so that crowds of people came to hear him and to be healed of their sicknesses."

Luk 5:15-16 (NIV)

"But despite Jesus' instructions, the report of his power spread even faster, and vast crowds came to hear him preach and to be healed of their diseases."

Luk 5:15-16 (NLT)

"For unto us was the gospel preached, as well as unto them: but the word preached did not profit them, not being mixed with faith in them that heard it."

Heb 4:2

"How then shall they call on him in whom they have not believed? and how shall they believe in him of whom they have not heard? and how shall they hear without a preacher?"

Rom 10:14

"The sower sows the word. And these are the ones along the path, where the word is sown: when they hear, Satan immediately comes and takes away the word that is sown in them. And these are the ones sown on rocky ground: the ones who, when they hear the word, immediately receive it with joy. And they have no root in themselves, but endure for a while; then, when tribulation or persecution arises on account of the word, immediately they fall away. And others are the ones sown among thorns. They are those who hear the word, but the cares of the world and the deceitfulness of riches and

the desires for other things enter in and choke
the word, and it proves unfruitful. But those that
were sown on the good soil are the ones who
hear the word and accept it and bear
fruit, thirtyfold and sixtyfold and a hundredfold."

Mar 4:14-20 (ESV)

"Now an angel of the Lord spoke to Philip,
saying, 'Arise and go toward the south along the
road which goes down from Jerusalem to Gaza.'
This is desert. So he arose and went. And
behold, a man of Ethiopia, a eunuch of great
authority under Candace the queen of the
Ethiopians, who had charge of all her treasury,
and had come to Jerusalem to worship, was
returning. And sitting in his chariot, he was
reading Isaiah the prophet. Then the Spirit said
to Philip, 'Go near and overtake this chariot.' So
Philip ran to him, and heard him reading the
prophet Isaiah, and said, 'Do you understand
what you are reading? And he said, 'How can I,
unless someone guides me?' And he asked Philip
to come up and sit with him. The place in the
Scripture which he read was this:

'He was led as a sheep to the slaughter;
And as a lamb before its shearer is silent,
So He opened not His mouth.
In His humiliation His justice was taken away,
And who will declare His generation?
For His life is taken from the earth.'

So the eunuch answered Philip and said, 'I ask you, of whom does the prophet say this, of himself or of some other man?' Then Philip opened his mouth, and beginning at this Scripture, preached Jesus to him. Now as they went down the road, they came to some water. And the eunuch said, 'See, here is water. What hinders me from being baptized?' Then Philip said, 'If you believe with all your heart, you may.' And he answered and said, 'I believe that Jesus Christ is the Son of God.' So he commanded the chariot to stand still. And both Philip and the eunuch went down into the water, and he baptized him. Now when they came up out of the water, the Spirit of the Lord caught Philip away, so that the eunuch saw him no more; and he went on his way rejoicing. But Philip was found at Azotus. And passing through, he preached in all the cities till he came to Caesarea."

Act 8:26-40 NKJV

I recently listened to a message by one of my favorite Bible teachers, Keith Moore of Moore Life Ministries (Faith Life Church Branson, MO and Sarasota, FL, https://www.moorelife.org/). I wanted to take from it and repackage it in this book. I couldn't.

I believe God told me to write this book and the one before it. However, Keith Moore is a spiritual mentor whom I have never met. I have quoted him in many of my books. I have seen him in person at a Kenneth Copeland convention. I highly revere his teachings.

Keith Moore is a graduate of Kenneth Hagin's Rhema Bible College. He was mentored and discipled by one of the greatest teachers of faith healing in the past generation, Kenneth Hagin. Keith Moore conducted Kenneth Hagin's healing school at Rhema.

If I were dying of an incurable disease or told by the doctors that there was "nothing more that they could do," I would travel to hear him preach on healing or consume his online content.

In other words, I would bet my life on his handling and teaching of the Word. In 1 The 2:4, Paul uses the phrase "entrusted with the gospel" pertaining to the call of God on his life. Keith Moore has been entrusted with the gospel, and I trust how he stewards and ministers it.

Below, I have included a link to part one of his series entitled "Hear and Be Healed." However, YouTube and other links get changed. If this link gets changed or fails to work for some reason, look up his ministry page and get anything that he has preached on the subject of healing, and follow him verse by verse in your Bible as he expounds upon the Word of God.

https://youtu.be/l8g7q4gBpB0

Again, I am not Keith Moore, and I can't bring what he brings to the body of Christ, nor am I supposed to. I can only bring what the Holy Spirit has given me. I believe what I share in this book complements what Keith Moore shared.

Sometimes, as Christians, we get stuck in an unfortunate place where we can only listen to one kind of Christian artist or music or to sermons from one denomination, race, etc. Please take what I have shared below and consider it along with Keith Moore's message.

(Please reread Heb 2:1 Mar 4:14-20 above)

Why do we need to hear and keep hearing the Word of God on healing or prosperity? Two reasons. One is because we can let the Word of God "slip in any area." We can lose sight of the revelation of the Word of God in any area.

The other reason is that we have an adversary. There is a devil at work, constantly trying to steal, choke, distract, persecute, and do anything to keep the Word of God from taking root and producing a harvest in our hearts. The Bible says the Word sown in our hearts can produce a harvest in varying degrees, thirty, sixty, or hundredfold. What causes the variation in the size of the harvest?

Some people have heard the Word and let it "slip" (Heb 2:1). Others have not guarded their hearts and allowed the enemy to steal it. Still others have placed a much higher priority on other desires and allowed these desires to choke off the harvest of the Word in their hearts.

When I thought of persecution for the Word, I first thought of the early Christians who were thrown to the lions. As a result, I almost ruled out that area of the enemy's current work. But then I believe the Holy Spirit made me think about the persecution we face from family, friends, and coworkers because of our faith or stance on healing, prosperity, etc.

I saved the stony grown/no root hearers of the Word for last on purpose. To explain it, I believe the Holy Spirit gave me a vision of how plants grow--

constant nurture and careful attention. You don't water a plant once and expect it to grow. Plants need the right amount of regular exposure to light and water to make their roots grow deeper and to make them strong.

We, our spirits, are like those plants. They need regular exposure to the light of the Word, the washing of the water of the Word (2 Cor 4:4, Eph 5:26). Faith comes by hearing and hearing and hearing the Word of God. Hearing the Word of God once in any area is not enough.

It's not enough because, as humans, we tend to let things slip. And because the enemy of our souls desires nothing more than to walk through the garden of our hearts and snatch up the Word that hasn't taken root and to sow desires for things that would choke off the harvest of the Word.

Our enemy would also like to bring harsh conditions into our garden, forms of persecution, or peer pressure that would cause us to stop giving constant and careful attention to the Word sown in the garden of our hearts.

How's the condition of the garden in your heart? How's your hearing pertaining to the Word of God in the area of healing?

Healing, God's Will Throughout the Ages

"For I am the Lord, I change not..."

Mal 3:6

"Jesus Christ the same yesterday, and today, and forever."

Heb 13:8

"When Jesus came down from the mountain, large crowds followed Him. Suddenly a leper came and knelt before Him, saying, "Lord, if You are willing, You can make me clean.' Jesus reached out His hand and touched the man. 'I am willing,' He said. 'Be clean!' And immediately his leprosy was cleansed...."

Mat 8:1-2

I spend a lot of time in this book talking about the work of Jesus, particularly in the area of healing. But if you look closely at the Old Testament, you will see that healing didn't begin with Jesus.

This is an important point because if I can get you to see that God's will was healing in the Old Testament and in the time of Jesus, then I can get you to understand that it is still His will today (see also the chapter entitled "He Healed Them All" in Vol I).

I wanted to try to use the fancy word dispensation, so I looked it up. That led me to a fancier word, dispensationalism, which spun off into the errors of dispensationalism. I didn't realize it was that complicated. I will try to take the concept as I imagined it and break it down the way I see it in Scripture.

In Scripture, I see a triune God working with man. In the Old Testament, I see God the Father speaking directly to men such as Adam, Moses, and Abraham and through the "word of the Lord" to the prophets (1Sa 3:21, 2Sa 3:24, 1Ki 13:2-18, Isa 39:5, Jer 1:2-4, etc.) and through the ministry of angels (Dan 10:5-9). I also see God the Father's expressed will concerning healing in the Old Testament.

In the New Testament, I see God the Son who put on flesh (Jhn 1:14, Phi 2:6-8), teaching, discipling, leading, and selecting leaders that would carry out His work when He left. In this book, I also detail Jesus carrying out the Father's will regarding healing.

Before He left, Jesus told the Apostles that He would send another Comforter (Jhn 16:14) and that it would be better that He left so that the Comforter could come (Jhn 16:7). That Comforter was God the Holy Ghost.

We see His operation on Earth mirroring everything that had been done by God the Father and God the Son. In the book of Acts and later chapters, we see the Holy Spirit working through men via gifts of healing and miracles.

In the simplest of terms, God, whether God the Father, God the Son, or God the Holy Ghost, has always been at work in the area of healing. Healing has always been God's promise and priority, and it makes sense that the three divine personalities would have the same priorities because They are all one.

Let's take a look at some Old Testament Scriptures that emphasize God's will for healing:

"Now when they came to Marah, they could not drink the waters of Marah, for they were bitter. Therefore the name of it was called Marah. And the people complained against Moses, saying, 'What shall we drink?' So he cried out to the Lord, and the Lord showed him a tree. When he cast it into the waters, the waters were made sweet. There He made a statute and an ordinance for them, and there He tested them, and said, 'If you diligently heed the voice of the Lord your God and do what is right in His sight, give ear to His commandments and keep all His statutes, I will put none of the diseases on you which I have brought on the Egyptians. For I am the Lord who heals you.'"

Exo 15:23-26 (NKJV)

"Praise the Lord, my soul; all my inmost being, praise his holy name. Praise the Lord, my soul, and forget not all his benefits—who forgives all your sins and heals all your diseases…"

Psa 103:1-3 (NIV)

"He also brought them out with silver and gold, and there was none feeble among His tribes. Egypt was glad when they departed, for the fear of them had fallen upon them."

Psa 105:37-38

"So you shall serve the LORD your God, and He will bless your bread and your water. And I will take sickness away from the midst of you. No

one shall suffer miscarriage or be barren in your
land; I will fulfill the number of your days."

Exo 23:25-26 (NKJV)

"And the LORD will take away from you all
sickness, and will afflict you with none of the
terrible diseases of Egypt which you have
known, but will lay them on all those who hate
you."

Deu 7:15 (NKJV)

"Do not be wise in your own eyes; Fear the LORD
and depart from evil. It will be health to your
flesh, And strength to your bones."

Pro 3:7-8 (NKJV)

"Now the blood shall be a sign for you on the
houses where you are. And when I see the
blood, I will pass over you; and the plague shall
not be on you to destroy you when I strike the
land of Egypt."

Exo 12:13 (NKJV)

"Because you have made the LORD, who is my
refuge, Even the Most High, your dwelling place,
No evil shall befall you, Nor shall any plague
come near your dwelling…"

Psa 91:9-10 (NKJV)

"Honour thy father and thy mother: that thy
days may be long upon the land which the LORD
thy God giveth thee."

Exo 20:12

"Ye shall walk in all the ways which the LORD
your God hath commanded you, that ye may
live, and that it may be well with you, and that
ye may prolong your days in the land which ye
shall possess."

Deu 5:33

"Many are the afflictions of the righteous: but
the LORD delivereth him out of them all."

Psa 34:19

"Then Aaron took it as Moses commanded, and ran into the midst of the assembly; and already the plague had begun among the people. So he put in the incense and made atonement for the people. And he stood between the dead and the living; so the plague was stopped."

Num 16:47-48

"The light of the eyes rejoices the heart, And a good report makes the bones healthy."

Pro 15:30

"Then your light shall break forth like the morning, Your healing shall spring forth speedily, And your righteousness shall go before you; The glory of the LORD shall be your rear guard."

Isa 58:8 (NKJV)

"But to you who fear My name the Sun of Righteousness shall arise with healing in His wings; and you shall go out And grow fat like stall-fed calves."

Mal 4:2 (NKJV)

"The days of our years are threescore years and ten; and if by reason of strength they be fourscore years, yet is their strength labour and sorrow; for it is soon cut off, and we fly away."

Psa 90:10

"My son, forget not my law; but let thine heart keep my commandments. For length of days, and long life, and peace, shall they add to thee."

Pro 3:1-2

"For by me thy days shall be multiplied, and the years of thy life shall be increased."

Pro 9:11

"Be not over much wicked, neither be thou foolish: why shouldest thou die before thy time?"

Ecc 7:17

"They shall not build, and another inhabit; they shall not plant, and another eat: for as the days of a tree are the days of my people, and mine elect shall long enjoy the work of their hands."

Isa 65:22

"I call heaven and earth to record this day against you, that I have set before you life and death, blessing and cursing: therefore choose life, that both thou and thy seed may live. That thou mayest love the LORD thy God, and that thou mayest obey his voice, and that thou mayest cleave unto him: for he is thy life, and the length of thy days: that thou mayest dwell in the land which the LORD sware unto thy fathers, to Abraham, to Isaac, and to Jacob, to give them."

Deu 30:19-20

"If ye walk in my statutes, and keep my commandments, and do them; for I will have respect unto you, and make you fruitful, and multiply you, and establish my covenant with you."

Lev 26:3, 9

"I shall not die, but live, And declare the works of the LORD."

Psa 118:17

"I will ransom them from the power of the grave; I will redeem them from death: O death, I will be thy plagues; O grave, I will be thy destruction: repentance shall be hid from mine eyes."

Hos 13:14

"For thus says the LORD to the house of Israel: 'Seek Me and live; but do not seek Bethel, Nor enter Gilgal, Nor pass over to Beersheba; for Gilgal shall surely go into captivity, and Bethel shall come to nothing. Seek the LORD and live, lest He break out like fire in the house of Joseph, and devour it, With no one to quench it in Bethel..."

Amo 5:4-6

"Honour thy father and thy mother: that thy days may be long upon the land which the LORD thy God giveth thee."

Exo 20:12

"Ye shall walk in all the ways which the LORD

your God hath commanded you, that ye may
live, and that it may be well with you, and that
ye may prolong your days in the land which ye
shall possess."

Deu 5:33

"...and that you may prolong your days in the
land which the LORD swore to give your fathers,
to them and their descendants, 'a land flowing
with milk and honey.'"

Deu 11:9 (NKJV)

"that your days and the days of your children
may be multiplied in the land of which the LORD
swore to your fathers to give them, like the days
of the heavens above the earth."

Deu 11:21 (NKJV)

"Even to your old age, I am He, And even to gray
hairs I will carry you! I have made, and I will
bear; Even I will carry, and will deliver you."

Isa 46:41

"And he died in a good old age, full of days,

riches, and honour: and Solomon his son reigned in his stead.”

Chr 29:28

“Thou shalt come to thy grave in a full age, like as a shock of corn cometh in his season.”

Job 5:26

“For a multitude of the people, even many of Ephraim, and Manasseh, Issachar, and Zebulun, had not cleansed themselves, yet did they eat the passover otherwise than it was written. But Hezekiah prayed for them, saying, The good LORD pardon every one that prepareth his heart to seek God, the LORD God of his fathers, though he be not cleansed according to the purification of the sanctuary. And the LORD hearkened to Hezekiah, and healed the people.

2Ch 30:18-20

“But he was wounded for our transgressions, he was bruised for our iniquities: the

chastisement of our peace was upon him; and
with his stripes we are healed."

Isa 53:5

"And it came to pass, when the king of Israel had
read the letter, that he rent his clothes, and
said, Am I God, to kill and to make alive, that this
man doth send unto me to recover a man of his
leprosy? wherefore consider, I pray you, and
see how he seeketh a quarrel against me. And it
was so, when Elisha the man of God had
heard that the king of Israel had rent his
clothes, that he sent to the king, saying,
Wherefore hast thou rent thy clothes? let him
come now to me, and he shall know that there
is a prophet in Israel. So Naaman came with his
horses and with his chariot, and stood at the
door of the house of Elisha. And Elisha sent a
messenger unto him, saying, Go and wash in
Jordan seven times, and thy flesh shall come
again to thee, and thou shalt be clean. But
Naaman was wroth, and went away, and
said, Behold, I thought, He will surely come
out to me, and stand, and call on the name of
the LORD his God, and strike his hand over the
place, and recover the leper. Are not Abana and
Pharpar, rivers of Damascus, better than all the

waters of Israel? may I not wash in them, and be
clean? So he turned and went away in a rage.
And his servants came near, and spake unto him,
and said, My father, if the prophet had
bid thee do some great thing, wouldest thou not
have done it? how much rather then, when he
saith to thee, Wash, and be clean? Then went he
down, and dipped himself seven times in
Jordan, according to the saying of the man of
God: and his flesh came again like unto the
flesh of a little child, and he was clean.

2 Ki 5:7-14

"And she went and did as Elijah said. And she
and he and her household ate for many
days. The jar of flour was not spent, neither did
the jug of oil become empty, according to the
word of the Lord that he spoke by Elijah. After
this the son of the woman, the mistress of the
house, became ill. And his illness was so severe
that there was no breath left in him. And she
said to Elijah, "What have you against me,
O man of God? You have come to me to bring
my sin to remembrance and to cause the death
of my son!" And he said to her, "Give me your
son." And he took him from her arms and carried
him up into the upper chamber where he
lodged, and laid him on his own bed. And he
cried to the Lord, "O Lord my God, have you

brought calamity even upon the widow with whom I sojourn, by killing her son?" Then he stretched himself upon the child three times and cried to the LORD, "O LORD my God, let this child's life come into him again." And the LORD listened to the voice of Elijah. And the life of the child came into him again, and he revived. And Elijah took the child and brought him down from the upper chamber into the house and delivered him to his mother. And Elijah said, "See, your son lives." And the woman said to Elijah, "Now I know that you are a man of God, and that the word of the LORD in your mouth is truth."

1 Ki 17:15-24

"When Elisha came into the house, he saw the child lying dead on his bed. So he went in and shut the door behind the two of them and prayed to the Lord. Then he went up and lay on the child, putting his mouth on his mouth, his eyes on his eyes, and his hands on his hands. And as he stretched himself upon him, the flesh of the child became warm. Then he got up again and walked once back and forth in the house, and went up and stretched himself upon him. The child sneezed seven times, and the child opened his eyes. Then he summoned Gehazi and

said, "Call this Shunammite." So he called her.
And when she came to him, he said, "Pick up
your son." She came and fell at his feet, bowing
to the ground. Then she picked up her son and
went out.

2 Ki 4:32-37

"And it came to pass, as they were burying a
man, that, behold, they spied a band of men;
and they cast the man into the sepulchre of
Elisha: and when the man was let down, and
touched the bones of Elisha, he revived, and
stood up on his feet."

2 Ki 13:21

The Old Testament is a written description of
God's covenant with Israel. They were His "chosen
people." The numerous Scriptures above show that
healing was a vital part of His covenant with them.

The Scriptural accounts of Elijah and Elisha read
like the gospels or the book of Acts. We see stories of
sick people being made well and the dead being
brought back to life. God used these men as conduits or
instruments of His healing power. It's the same pattern
seen in the apostles selected by Jesus and later in men

like Stephen and Philip, whom the Holy Ghost chose through the apostles.

In the New Testament, when we receive Christ as Savior, we come into covenant with God. The Bible says in Heb 8:1-13 that we, as New Testament believers and covenant members, have a better covenant:

"Now of the things which we have spoken this is the sum: We have such an high priest, who is set on the right hand of the throne of the Majesty in the heavens; A minister of the sanctuary, and of the true tabernacle, which the Lord pitched, and not man. For every high priest is ordained to offer gifts and sacrifices: wherefore it is of necessity that this man have somewhat also to offer. For if he were on Earth, he should not be a priest, seeing that there are priests that offer gifts according to the law: Who serve unto the example and shadow of heavenly things, as Moses was admonished of God when he was about to make the tabernacle: for, See, saith he, that thou make all things according to the pattern shewed to thee in the mount. But now hath he obtained a more excellent ministry, by how much also he is the mediator of a better covenant, which was established upon better promises. For if that first covenant had been faultless, then should no place have been sought for the second. In that he saith, A new covenant, he hath made the first old. Now that which decayeth and waxeth old is ready to vanish away."

I end this chapter with a request. Reflect on the number of healing scriptures in the Old Testament and ask yourself: If healing was an integral part of the old covenant and we have a new and better covenant, why wouldn't it be part of it?

Jesus went about "healing and doing good" (Act 10:38). It demonstrated that God's will for healing was still part of the covenant promises. Jesus said I came to do the will of Him who sent me (Jhn 6:38). In later chapters, I will show that God the Holy Ghost continued this work after Jesus departed. Truly, healing was and is God's will throughout the ages.

One, Twelve, Seventy-Two

"He who sins is of the devil, for the devil has sinned from the beginning. For this purpose the Son of God was manifested, that He might destroy the works of the devil."

1 Jh 3:8 (NKJV)

"Jesus went throughout Galilee, teaching in their synagogues, proclaiming the good news of the kingdom, and <u>healing every disease and sickness</u> among the people. News about him spread all over Syria, and people brought to him <u>all who were ill with various diseases</u>, those suffering severe pain, the demon-possessed, those having seizures, and the paralyzed; <u>and he healed them</u>. Large crowds from Galilee, the Decapolis, Jerusalem, Judea and the region across the Jordan followed him."

*underlining added for emphasis

Mat 4:23-25 (NIV)

"At sunset, <u>the people brought to Jesus all who had various kinds of sickness</u>, and laying his hands on each one, <u>he healed them</u>. Moreover, demons came out of many people, shouting, "You are the Son of God!" But he rebuked them and would not allow them to speak, because they knew he was the Messiah."

*underlining added for emphasis

Luk 4:40-41 (NIV)

"How God anointed Jesus of Nazareth with the Holy Ghost and with power, and how He went about doing good and <u>healing all</u> who were oppressed by the devil, for God was with Him."

*underlining added for emphasis

Act 10:38

1 Jhn 3:8 says that Jesus was manifested, i.e., "made visible," "made known," or "exposed to view" (Strong's Concordance) (Blue Letter Bible, n.d.) to destroy the works of the devil. If Jesus had a mission statement or a statement of purpose, part of it would be to destroy the works of the devil, the one who "sinned from the beginning." In several places in

Scripture, Jesus says He only did the will of the Father that sent Him.

> "I can of mine own self do nothing: as I hear, I judge and my judgment is just; because I seek not mine
> own will, but the will of the Father which hath sent me."

Jhn 5:30

> "Jesus said to them, 'My food is to do the will of Him who sent Me, and to finish His work.'"

Jhn 4:34 (NKJV)

> "For I have come down from heaven not to do my will but to do the will of him who sent me. And this is the will of him who sent me, that I shall lose none of all those he has given me, but raise them up at the last day. For my Father's will is that everyone who looks to the Son and believes in him shall have eternal life, and I will raise them up at the last day."

Jhn 6:38-40 (NIV)

"Most assuredly, I say to you, he who believes in
Me, the works that I do he will do also; and
greater *works* than these he will do, because I go
to My Father. And whatever you ask in My
name, that I will do, that the Father may
be glorified in the Son. If you ask anything in My
name, I will do *it.*"

Jhn 14:12

If we follow Jesus' life in the gospels, we can see
that healing was part of His mission and one of His
priorities. One of the greatest proofs of the priority
Jesus placed on healing is seen in what He told others to
do. If we look at Jesus' instructions to the apostles and
the "seventy-two," we see that healing was one of the
highest priorities.

Sending Out the Twelve

"Then He called His twelve disciples together
and gave them power and authority over all
demons, <u>and to cure diseases</u>. He sent them to
preach the kingdom of God and to heal the
sick. And He said to them, 'Take nothing for the
journey, neither staffs nor bag nor bread nor

money; and do not have two tunics apiece. Whatever house you enter, stay there, and from there depart. And whoever will not receive you, when you go out of that city, shake off the very dust from your feet as a testimony against them.' So they departed and went through the towns, preaching the gospel and <u>healing everywhere</u>."

*underlining added for emphasis

Luk 9:1-6 (NKJV)

"And through the hands of the apostles many signs and wonders were done among the people. And they were all with one accord in Solomon's Porch. Yet none of the rest dared join them, but the people esteemed them highly. And believers were increasingly added to the Lord, multitudes of both men and women, so that they brought the sick out into the streets and laid them on beds and couches, that at least the shadow of Peter passing by might fall on some of them. Also a multitude gathered from the surrounding cities to Jerusalem, bringing sick people and those who were tormented by unclean spirits, and they were all healed."

Act 5:12-16 (NKJV)

Jesus Sends Out the Seventy-Two

"After this the Lord appointed seventy-two
and sent them on ahead of him, two by two, into
every town and place where he himself was
about to go. And he said to them, 'The harvest is
plentiful, but the laborers are few. Therefore
pray earnestly to the Lord of the harvest to send
out laborers into his harvest. Go your
way; behold, I am sending you out as lambs in
the midst of wolves. Carry no moneybag, no
knapsack, no sandals, and greet no one on the
road. Whatever house you enter, first
say, 'Peace be to this house!' And if a son of
peace is there, your peace will rest upon him.
But if not, it will return to you. And remain in the
same house, eating and drinking what they
provide, for the laborer deserves his wages. Do
not go from house to house. Whenever you
enter a town and they receive you, eat what is
set before you. <u>Heal the sick</u> in it and say to
them, 'The kingdom of God has come near to
you.'"

*underlining added for emphasis

Luk 10:1-9 (NKJV)

"Afterward he appeared unto the eleven as they sat at meat, and upbraided them with their unbelief and hardness of heart, because they believed not them which had seen him after he was risen. And he said unto them, Go ye into all the world, and preach the gospel to every creature. He that believeth and is baptized shall be saved; but he that believeth not shall be damned. And these signs shall follow them that believe; In my name shall they cast out devils; they shall speak with new tongues; They shall take up serpents; and if they drink any deadly thing, it shall not hurt them; they shall <u>lay hands on the sick, and they shall recover.</u> So then after the Lord had spoken unto them, he was received up into heaven, and sat on the right hand of God. And they went forth, and preached every where, the Lord working with them, and confirming the word with signs following. Amen."

*underlining added for emphasis

Mar 16:14-20

2 Tim 3:16-17 says, "All scripture is given by inspiration of God, and is profitable for doctrine, for reproof, for correction, for instruction in righteousness:

That the man of God may be perfect, thoroughly furnished unto all good works." If we let Scripture inform our doctrine, we steer clear of error.

There are church traditions that limit God's healing power to Jesus or His disciples. Jesus healed others as a man empowered by God. So did the apostles, and so did the seventy-two.

After He died on the cross, Jesus appeared and said that those who "believe" would also lay hands on the sick and that they'd recover. Those who believe are a far larger group than the twelve and the seventy-two. Further, it is implied that these believers would also make healing a priority.

Healing is part of the "greater works" Jesus promised we'd do because He was going to the Father (Jhn 14:12). This healing power manifests through Holy Spirit-enabled people who were to come after the twelve and the seventy-two. The work of the Holy Spirit to heal is the next chapter's subject.

Gifts of Healing and Miracles

"The priests the Levites, and all the tribe of
Levi, shall have no part nor inheritance with
Israel: they shall eat the offerings of the
LORD made by fire, and his inheritance.
Therefore shall they have no
inheritance among their brethren: the
LORD is their inheritance, as he hath said unto
them. And this shall be the priest's due from the
people, from them that offer a
sacrifice, whether it be ox or sheep; and they
shall give unto the priest the shoulder, and the
two cheeks, and the maw. The firstfruit also of
thy corn, of thy wine, and of thine oil, and the
first of the fleece of thy sheep, shalt thou
give him. For the LORD thy God hath chosen him
out of all thy tribes, to stand to minister in the
name of the LORD, him and his sons for ever."

Deu 18:1-5

"The LORD thy God will raise up unto thee a
Prophet from the midst of thee, of thy
brethren, like unto me; unto him ye shall
hearken...I will raise them up a Prophet from

among their brethren, like unto thee, and will
put my words in his mouth; and he shall
speak unto them all that I shall command him.
And it shall come to pass, that whosoever will
not hearken unto my words which he shall
speak in my name, I will require it of him."

Deu 18:15, 18-19

"And I will give you pastors according to mine
heart, which shall feed you with knowledge and
understanding."

Jer 3:15

In the Old Testament, we see many examples of
God raising leaders up to guide, minister, and intervene
on behalf of His chosen people. We see people
identified by God and anointed to be priests, prophets,
and kings (Saul, David). We also see leaders like
Abraham, Moses, Joseph, Esther, and Daniel. These men
and women were chosen by God and empowered by
the Spirit of God to perform leadership tasks in
nurturing, guiding, teaching, and protecting the children
of Israel.

"Samson went down to Timnah together with his
father and mother. As they approached the
vineyards of Timnah, suddenly a young lion
came roaring toward him. The Spirit of
the Lord came powerfully upon him so that he
tore the lion apart with his bare hands as he
might have torn a young goat. But he told
neither his father nor his mother what he had
done."

Jud 14:5-6

"And the Spirit of God came upon Azariah the
son of Oded: And he went out to meet Asa, and
said unto him, Hear ye me, Asa, and all Judah
and Benjamin; The LORD is with you, while ye be
with him; and if ye seek him, he will be found of
you; but if ye forsake him, he will forsake
you. Now for a long season Israel hath
been without the true God, and without a
teaching priest, and without law."

2 Chr 15:1-3

"Then Samuel took the horn of oil and anointed
him in the midst of his brothers; and the Spirit of
the LORD came upon David from that day
forward. So Samuel arose and went to Ramah."

1 Sam 16:13

"Then upon Jahaziel the son of Zechariah, the
son of Benaiah, the son of Jeiel, the son of
Mattaniah, a Levite of the sons of Asaph, came
the Spirit of the LORD in the midst of the
congregation; And he said, Hearken ye, all
Judah, and ye inhabitants of Jerusalem, and thou
king Jehoshaphat, Thus saith the LORD unto you,
Be not afraid nor dismayed by reason of this
great multitude; for the battle is not yours, but
God's."

2 Ch 20:14-15

"Then the Spirit of the LORD came on me, and
he told me to say: 'This is what the LORD says:
That is what you are saying, you leaders in Israel,
but I know what is going through your mind.'"

Eze 11:5 NIV

"So Moses went out and relayed to the people
the words of the LORD, and he gathered seventy
of the elders of the people and had them stand
around the tent. Then the LORD came down in

the cloud and spoke to him, and He took some
of the Spirit that was on Moses and placed that
Spirit on the seventy elders. As the
Spirit rested on them, they prophesied— but
they never did so again."

Num 11:24-25

God loved His chosen people so much that He
handpicked men and women leaders to guide, teach,
lead, nurture, deliver, and rule. These handpicked
leaders were anointed or empowered by the Spirit of
God upon them to prophesy, to deliver, to interpret
dreams (Dan 2:27), to have divine favor (Est 2:17, Gen
39:4-6), and to heal (1Ki 17:17-24). But what about us?

The Bible says of us that, "God so loved the
world, that he gave His only begotten Son..." (Jhn 3:16).
It stands to reason that if God loves us as much as He
did His chosen people in the Old Testament that He
would identify and anoint leaders for us. That is
precisely what He did. We see leaders selected by God
and anointed by the Spirit of the Lord in the New
Testament.

"Wherefore he saith, When he ascended up on
high, he led captivity captive, and gave gifts unto

men....And he gave some, apostles; and some, prophets; and some, evangelists; and some, pastors and teachers; For the perfecting of the saints, for the work of the ministry, for the edifying of the body of Christ: Till we all come in the unity of the faith, and of the knowledge of the Son of God, unto a perfect man, unto the measure of the stature of the fulness of Christ: That we henceforth be no more children, tossed to and fro, and carried about with every wind of doctrine, by the sleight of men, and cunning craftiness, whereby they lie in wait to deceive; But speaking the truth in love, may grow up into him in all things, which is the head, even Christ: From whom the whole body fitly joined together and compacted by that which every joint supplieth, according to the effectual working in the measure of every part, maketh increase of the body unto the edifying of itself in love."

Eph 4:8, 12-16

"And God hath set some in the church: first apostles, secondarily prophets, thirdly teachers, after that miracle workers, then those with gifts of healing, helpers, administrators, and those with diversity of tongues."

1 Cor 12:28

"Now there are diversities of gifts, but the same
Spirit. And there are differences of
administrations, but the same Lord. And there
are diversities of operations, but it is the same
God which worketh all in all. But the
manifestation of the Spirit is given to every man
to profit withal. For to one is given by the Spirit
the word of wisdom; to another the word of
knowledge by the same Spirit; To another faith
by the same Spirit; to another the gifts of healing
by the same Spirit; To another the working of
miracles; to another prophecy; to another
discerning of spirits; to another divers kinds of
tongues; to another the interpretation of
tongues: But all these worketh that one and the
selfsame Spirit, dividing to every man severally
as he will."

1 Cor 12:4-11

"And in these days came prophets from Jerusale
m unto Antioch. And there stood
up one of them named Agabus, and
signified by the Spirit that there should
be great dearth throughout all the

world: which came to pass in the days
of Claudius Caesar."

Act 11:27-28

"Now there were in the church that was at
Antioch certain prophets and teachers;
as Barnabas, and Simeon that was
called Niger, and Lucius of Cyrene, and Manaen,
which had been brought up with Herod the
tetrarch, and Saul."

Act 13:1

"And there was one Anna, a prophetess, the
daughter of Phanuel, of the tribe of
Aser: she was of a great age, and had
lived with an husband seven years from her
virginity;"

Luk 2:36

In the New Testament, in Ephesians 4, God calls
apostles, prophets, evangelists, pastors, and teachers
"gifts." The giving of leaders by God was a concept also
seen in the Old Testament. In Exo 3:9-19 we see God
sending Moses in response to the cry of His people: "I

have indeed heard the cry of my people, and I see how the Egyptians are oppressing them. Now I am sending you to the king of Egypt so that you can lead my people out of his country." In 1Sa 8:1-22 we see God give Israel a king, King Saul, and later King David (1Sa 16:1-13).

Some of these Ephesians 4 gifts and their operation are not new. The Old Testament is full of references to prophets. Even Abraham is referred to as a prophet in Gen 20:7:

> "Now therefore restore the man his wife; for he is a prophet, and he shall pray for thee, and thou shalt live: and if thou restore her not, know thou that thou shalt surely die, thou, and all that are thine."

Though I am not very familiar with the operation of pastors in the Old Testament, relative to the function of the priests, they are mentioned in the Old Testament. Jer 3:15 says, "And I will give you pastors according to mine heart, which shall feed you with knowledge and understanding." According to the Strong's Concordance, The Hebrew word rāʿâ, used for pastors in Jer 3:15, occurs 173 times in the Old Testament.

"KJV Translation Count — Total: 173x

The KJV translates Strong's H7462 in the
following manner: feed (75x), shepherd (63x),
pastor (8x), herdmen (7x), keep (3x), companion
(2x), broken (1x), company (1x), devour (1x), eat
(1x), entreateth (1x), miscellaneous (10x)."

(Blue Letter Bible, n.d.)

According to the following Scriptures in
Jeremiah, these Old Testament "pastors" seem to have
a function similar to pastors in the New Testament (feed
the sheep, shepherd, keep the sheep):

"LORD, I have not abandoned my job as a
shepherd for your people. I have not urged you
to send disaster. You have heard everything I've
said."

Jer 17:16 NLT

"The priests said not, Where is the LORD? and
they that handle the law knew me not:
the pastors also transgressed against me, and
the prophets prophesied by Baal, and
walked after things that do not profit."

Jer 2:8

"And I will give you pastors according to mine heart, which shall feed you with knowledge and understanding."

Jer 3:15

"For the pastors are become brutish, and have not sought the LORD: therefore they shall not prosper, and all their flocks shall be scattered."

Jer 10:21

"Woe be unto the pastors that destroy and scatter the sheep of my pasture! saith the LORD. Therefore thus saith the LORD God of Israel against the pastors that feed my people; Ye have scattered my flock, and driven them away, and have not visited them: behold, I will visit upon you the evil of your doings, saith the LORD."

Jer 23:1-2

The Ephesians 4 list of gifts God gave us includes apostles, prophets, evangelists, pastors, and teachers.

The Bible says that the body of Christ is edified or built up through these gifts. Further, Eph 4:12-16 says that God uses these gifts to perfect or mature the saints, keep them from being deceived by false doctrine, and mold them into a unified body of Christ, an entity in which every part works together effectively in love.

I believe the Holy Spirit working through these gifts (commonly called the five-fold ministry gifts: apostles, prophets, evangelists, pastors, and teachers) accomplishes God's will for the body of Christ in Eph 4:12-16. In the passage below, we see Paul exhorting Timothy to preach and to "do the work of an evangelist."

"I charge thee therefore before God, and the
Lord Jesus Christ, who shall judge the
quick and the dead at his appearing and his
kingdom; Preach the word; be instant in
season, out of season; reprove, rebuke, exhort
with all longsuffering and doctrine. For the
time will come when they will not endure sound
doctrine; but after their own lusts shall they
heap to themselves teachers, having
itching ears; And they shall turn
away their ears from the truth, and shall be
turned unto fables. But watch thou in all

things, endure afflictions, do the work of an evangelist, make full proof of thy ministry."

2 Ti 4:1-5

The Ephesians 4 list, however, is not an exhaustive list of the leadership gifts God gave us in the New Testament. 1 Cor 12:28 talks of other gifts "set in the church" by God. Recently, the Holy Spirit showed me in this verse that "miracle workers" and "those with gifts of healing" were set in the Church (capitalized to represent the Church at large or the entire body of Christ) to accomplish His will. These people are mentioned just after apostles, prophets, and teachers. They are mentioned ahead of or alongside, if you prefer, those with administrative and helping gifts.

As it pertains to healing, this is such a powerful revelation. I had always thought of gifts of healing as something that operated by the Holy Spirit according to His will (1 Cor 12:11 NLT: "It is the one and only Spirit who distributes all these gifts.) He alone decides which gift each person should have." And what I believed was not inaccurate; it was just incomplete. The revelation I'd had of healing and miracles was that of some less frequently manifested gift of the Spirit.

But in these Scriptures, the Holy Spirit revealed that healing and miracles were so important to God that He planned them to be part of the Church's structure and operation. God intended for people who work miracles and have gifts of healing to be present in the Church right along with apostles, prophets, teachers, evangelists, administrators, helpers, those who interpret tongues, etc.

What a wonderful revelation! It was plainly written in Scripture, but I had not seen it. God set gifts of healing and miracles in the Church just like He did the Eph 4 gifts of apostles, pastors, teachers, evangelists, prophets, and those with gifts of administration and helping gifts.

I want to examine two New Testament men who operated in the Eph 4 and 1 Cor 12 gifts. Those men are Stephen and Phillip.

"Then the twelve summoned the multitude of the disciples and said, 'It is not desirable that we should leave the word of God and serve tables. Therefore, brethren, seek out from among you seven men of good reputation, full of the Holy Spirit and wisdom, whom we may appoint over this business; but we will give ourselves continually to prayer and to the ministry of the word.' And the saying pleased the whole multitude. And they chose Stephen, a man full of faith and the Holy Spirit, and Philip, Prochorus, Nicanor, Timon, Parmenas, and Nicolas, a proselyte from Antioch, whom

they set before the apostles; and when they had
prayed, they laid hands on them. Then the word
of God spread, and the number of the disciples
multiplied greatly in Jerusalem, and a great
many of the priests were obedient to the faith.
And Stephen, full of faith and power, did
great wonders and signs among the people."

Act 6:2-8 (NKJV)

"Then Philip went down to the city of Samaria
and preached Christ to them. And the multitudes
with one accord heeded the things spoken by
Philip, hearing and seeing the miracles which he
did. For unclean spirits, crying with a loud voice,
came out of many who were possessed; and
many who were paralyzed and lame were
healed. And there was great joy in that city."

Act 8:5-8 (NKJV)

"On the next day we who were Paul's
companions departed and came to Caesarea,
and entered the house of Philip the
evangelist, who was one of the seven, and
stayed with him."

Act 21:8 (NKJV)

We have seen prophets and pastors in both the Old and New Testaments. What about miracle workers and those operating with gifts of healing? Were those gifts seen in operation in the Old Testament? Yes!

God's leaders in the Old Testament performed miracles (Moses, Daniel, Elijah, Elisha, Sampson, Joshua, etc.) and healings (Elijah (1Ki 17:17-24), Elisha (2Ki 4:18-37)). *See Appendix A, "42 Miracles and Wonders Performed by Moses." The apostles and the seventy-two sent out by Jesus performed miracles and healings.

If God's leaders in both the Old and New Testament performed miracles and healings, why wouldn't we expect the same today? The same Holy Spirit that empowered the Old and New Testament saints is present to move and operate today.

Why do we in the body of Christ so readily acknowledge and expect the Church to have apostles, prophets, pastors, teachers, evangelists, administrators, and helpers but not miracle workers and those operating with gifts of healing? How has the Church come to diminish the place and the contribution of these gifts compared to others that God "set in the church?"

I believe the devil has attacked and purposely suppressed the revelation of these gifts. Before I describe how the devil has done this, I'd like to share why I believe he has done so.

As I considered the devil's motivations, I believe the Holy Spirit made me think about Jesus and why the large crowds followed Him. I believe Jesus attracted large crowds because of the many miracles and healings he performed.

Acts 10:38 says, "God anointed Jesus of Nazareth with the Holy Ghost and with power, and how He went about doing good and healing all who were oppressed by the devil, for God was with Him." Crowds of people assembled to see Jesus perform a miracle or in hopes of being healed. Jesus' preaching was intertwined with his performance of miracles. Everyone who came to see a miracle or receive healing heard Jesus' teaching.

In a sense, revival, in the form of a willingness to hear the gospel, was sparked by the healings and miracles Jesus performed. Perhaps the Church no longer sees great revivals because of the lack of healings and miracles. For my Charismatic and Pentecostal readers, yes, great revival can happen just by a mighty outpouring of the presence of the Holy Spirit. Still, the pattern laid out by Jesus is irrefutable.

If it is true, and I believe I have shown that it is, healings and miracles can lead to revival and people coming to believe in the Lordship of Jesus Christ, then it would be in Satan's best interest to stop it. How does he try to stop it? There are several ways the Scriptures show us:

"The thief does not come except to steal, and to kill, and to destroy. I have come that they may have life, and that they may have it more abundantly."

Jhn 10:10 (NKJV)

"The god of this age has blinded the minds of unbelievers, so that they cannot see the light of the gospel that displays the glory of Christ, who is the image of God."

2 Cor 4:4 (NIV)

"My people are destroyed for lack of knowledge: because thou hast rejected knowledge,..."

Hos 4:6

"The sower soweth the word. And these are they by the way side, where the word is sown; but when they have heard, Satan cometh immediately, and taketh away the word that was sown in their hearts. And these are they likewise which are sown on stony ground; who, when they have heard the word, immediately receive it with gladness; And have no root in themselves, and so endure but for a time: afterward, when affliction or persecution ariseth for the word's sake, immediately they are offended. And these are they which are sown among thorns; such as hear the word, And the cares of this world, and the deceitfulness of riches, and the lusts of other things entering in, choke the word, and it becometh unfruitful. And these are they which are sown on good ground; such as hear the word, and receive it, and bring forth fruit, some thirtyfold, some sixty, and some an hundred."

Mar 4:14-20

"Making the word of God of none effect through your tradition, which ye have delivered: and many such like things do ye."

Mar 7:13

From the Scriptures above, we can see that Satan's job is to "steal, kill, and destroy," while Jesus' mission is to bring abundant life. Satan steals abundance from us using the following means referenced in the Scriptures: blindness, lack of knowledge, choking the word, lust for other things, the deceitfulness of riches, and religious tradition.

If Satan can blind you to the truth about miracles and healing and their importance to God, you won't be healed. If Satan can keep you ignorant of the many Scriptures that emphasize healing as a core part of the gospel, the good news of Jesus Christ, you will be destroyed for lack of knowledge. If Satan can get you to accept religious traditions that say healings and miracles have passed away or they are not for all, despite the Bible saying God set these gifts in the Church, you won't benefit from these gifts.

"Jesus Christ is the same yesterday, today, and forever."

Heb 13:8 (NKJV)

"For I am the Lord, I change not; therefore ye sons of Jacob are not consumed."

Mal 3:6

"For this purpose the Son of God was manifested, that He might destroy the works of the devil."

1 Jh 3:8

"...how God anointed Jesus of Nazareth with the
Holy Spirit and with power, who went about
doing good and healing all who were oppressed
by the devil, for God was with Him."

Act 10:38

It was God's will to do miracles and healings and
prevent sickness in the Old Testament. He sent Jesus to
destroy the works of the devil (e.g., sickness) in the New
Testament. Jesus did this as The Holy Spirit empowered
him. Jesus raised up other leaders who, by the power of
the Spirit, did similar things in line with Jesus'
exhortation:

"Most assuredly, I say to you, he who believes in
Me, the works that I do he will do also; and
greater works than these he will do, because I go
to My Father."

Jhn 14:12 (NKJV)

"And it happened that the father of Publius lay
sick of a fever and dysentery. Paul went in to
him and prayed, and he laid his hands on him
and healed him. So when this was done, the rest

of those on the island who had diseases also came and were healed."

Act 28:8-9 (NKJV)

"And in Lystra a certain man without strength in his feet was sitting, a cripple from his mother's womb, who had never walked. This man heard Paul speaking. Paul, observing him intently and seeing that he had faith to be healed, said with a loud voice, 'Stand up straight on your feet!' And he leaped and walked."

Act 14:8-10

Jesus selected leaders that discipled other leaders, who, by the power of the Holy Spirit, did miracles and healings. God set healings and miracles in the Church. His will has not changed. In the next chapter, we will look at some modern-day examples of men and women who operated in the gifts of miracles and healing, and we will look at what the devil has done to steal and destroy the operation of these gifts in the body of Christ.

Modern-Day Healers and Miracle Workers

"Verily, verily, I say unto you, He that believeth on me, the works that I do shall he do also; and greater works than these shall he do; because I go unto my Father."

Jhn 14:12 (KJV)

"And these signs will follow those
who believe: In My name they will cast out demons; they will speak with new
tongues; they will take up serpents; and if they drink anything deadly, it will by no means hurt them; they will lay hands on the sick, and they will recover."

Mar 16:17-20 (NKJV)

"And God was doing extraordinary miracles by the hands of Paul, so that even handkerchiefs or aprons that had touched his skin were carried away to the sick, and their diseases left them and the evil spirits came out of them."

Act 19:11 (ESV)

"God forbid: yea, let God be true, but every man a liar; as it is written, That thou mightest be justified in thy sayings, and mightest overcome when thou art judged."

Rom 3:4 (KJV)

I have struggled mightily to finish this chapter. Writing it was the most significant obstacle I had to overcome to finish the book. I struggled because I didn't know how to disprove the naysayers who say that the great men and women who performed healing miracles after the time of the twelve apostles were all false teachers.

I have studied the lives and read the books of some of these great men and women of God, and my heart ached, and my anger burned against those who would proclaim that their work under the power and direction of the Holy Spirit was false.

Recently, I believe the Holy Spirit gave me the answer to my dilemma. It, as answers from God typically are, was simple yet profound. The response to the naysayers can be found in the words of Jesus.

Jesus said that we, as believers, would do greater works than the works He performed on earth.

He wasn't just talking to the twelve apostles. Jesus said that there would be signs that follow those who believe. I have shown throughout this book that in the Old and New Testament, healings were performed outside of those performed by Jesus and the Twelve.

I have detailed in Scripture after Scripture the will and the power of God to heal throughout the Bible. The power of God that healed in the Old Testament, that flowed through Jesus, the Twelve, and Paul, is still active and available today.

That power has a name. It is the Holy Ghost. The Holy Spirit that moved upon the face of the waters at creation (Gen 1:2) and raised Christ from the dead (Rom 6:10-11) still moves today. The Holy Spirit moves and manifests in gifts of healing, miracles, and words of knowledge. The power of the Holy Spirit is manifested or activated by faith today just as it was manifested through Jesus and the Twelve.

Jesus is the "same yesterday, today and forever." The Holy Spirit is the same. How is it, then, that the operation of the Holy Spirit in modern times gets to be viewed with such disbelief? How did it come to be that the "healers" and "miracle workers" of my grandparents, parents, and my lifetime come to be thought of as frauds, charlatans, and false teachers?

In my research for this book, I ran across a commentary on Smith Wigglesworth, one of the greatest faith healers and miracle workers of his or any recent generation. I'd like to walk through the points found in the commentary in hopes of dismantling and dispelling the biblical inaccuracies contained in it.

"Of course, Jesus healed many people as evidence of His deity and power. And the twelve apostles were given the gift of healing as confirmation of their message to the world. But there are no apostles today, and those who claim to fill that role or to have the power of an apostle are deceivers. Today's 'faith healers,' like their protégé Smith Wigglesworth, perform their 'miracles' only in carefully organized meetings and on a stage they control. None of them are walking through hospitals healing everyone as they go.

Smith Wigglesworth taught several false doctrines:

• All sickness is proof of the presence of the devil. This leaves no room for God's purposes in suffering (2 Corinthians 1:8–9; Hebrews 12:6).
• Illness and disease are linked to personal sin. This ignores Jesus' teaching on the subject (John 9:1–3).

• It is always God's will to heal a person physically. Paul's testimony teaches the contrary, that it is not always God's will to heal us in this life (2 Corinthians 12:7–10).
• If a person is not healed, the blame lies in that person's lack of faith. This overlooks the fact that Jesus once healed a man who had no faith at all (John 5:1–9).

Given all the false teaching from Smith Wigglesworth, we conclude that he was a false teacher, regardless of whatever popularity he enjoyed and whatever shows of power he may have included in his act." (Got Questions, n.d.)

Commentary Inaccuracies detailed:

- *"the twelve apostles were given the gift of healing as confirmation of their message to the world."*
    o In Luke 9:1-2 (KJV): "Then he called his twelve disciples together, and gave them power and authority over all devils, and to cure diseases. And he sent them to preach the kingdom of God, and to heal the sick."
    o While it is true that Jesus gave the twelve apostles the power to heal the sick, he gave the same power to the seventy-two.

- o   Luk 10:1, 9: "After this the Lord appointed seventy-two and sent them on ahead of him, two by two, into every town and place where he himself was about to go… Whenever you enter a town and they receive you, eat what is set before you. Heal the sick in it and say to them, 'The kingdom of God has come near to you.'" Later, the Apostle Paul (Acts chapters 14, 20) and Philip (Acts Chapter 8) also performed healing miracles.
- *"This leaves no room for God's purposes in suffering"* (2 Corinthians 1:8–9; Hebrews 12:6).
    - o 2 Cor 1:8-9 (ESV): "For we do not want you to be unaware, brothers, of the affliction we experienced in Asia. For we were so utterly burdened beyond our strength that we despaired of life itself. Indeed, we felt that we had received the sentence of death. But that was to make us rely not on ourselves but on God who raises the dead."
    - o The author of the commentary presumes sickness is included in "God's purposes in suffering" and in the "affliction" Paul suffered. The word affliction in this Scripture is thlîpsis. None of the definitions or uses of this word refer to sickness or disease: "The KJV translates Strong's G2347 in the following manner:

tribulation (21x), affliction (17x), trouble (3x), anguish (1x), persecution (1x), burdened (1x) , to be afflicted (with G1519) (1x). Outline of Biblical Usage: a pressing, pressing together, pressure metaphor, oppression, affliction, tribulation, distress, straits" (Blue Letter Bilble, n.d.)

- o Hebrews 12:6 (ESV): "For the Lord disciplines the one he loves, and chastises every son whom he receives."
- o The author of this commentary presumes, with no Scriptural evidence, that God disciplines those He loves with sickness and disease. What a horrible assault on the character of God! If we study the lives of some of those with whom God had a close relationship, such as Moses, Abraham, and David, men who made terrible mistakes, we NEVER see God chastising them with sickness and disease. Jesus rebuked the disciples and even told Peter, "Get thee behind me, Satan," but never chastised them with sickness and disease. One of the ways the Bible says God corrects us is through the Word of God. 2 Tim 3:16-17 says, "All scripture is given by inspiration of God, and is profitable for doctrine, for reproof, for correction, for instruction in righteousness: That the man of God may be perfect, thoroughly furnished unto all good works."

- *"This ignores Jesus' teaching on the subject* (John 9:1–3)."
  - o Jhn 9:1–3 (ESV): "As he passed by, he saw a man blind from birth. And his disciples asked him, "Rabbi, who sinned, this man or his parents, that he was born blind?" Jesus answered, "It was not that this man sinned, or his parents, but that the works of God might be displayed in him."
  - o The author of the commentary and many others have wrongly interpreted this Scripture to mean that the man's blindness was the work of God or that God's will was that this man be blind. I contend that the "work" that God wanted to be "displayed" in him was God's miraculous power over blindness! I contend that this man was born blind and was there to encounter Jesus at the time that he did so that God could demonstrate that the power of God to heal is greater than blindness.
  - o Further, if it were God's will for the man to be blind, why would Jesus go around undoing the work and will of God and working against His purposes in the earth? Well, the answer is He wouldn't. In fact, the Bible says in 1 Jhn 3:8, "For this purpose the Son of God was manifested, that he might destroy the works of the devil." Jesus destroyed the work of

blindness in the man because it was the work
of the devil and not the work of the Father.
- o The author of the commentary seems to imply
  that sickness can't be linked to personal sin.
  In 1 John chapter five, Jesus tells the man
  who had been healed of an infirmity after 38
  years, "See, you have been made well. Sin no
  more, lest a worse thing come upon you."
  The man had an infirmity that crippled him
  for 38 years, yet Jesus tells him that
  something worse could come upon him if he
  sinned again. This seems to be consistent
  with Eph 4:27 (KJV) "Neither give place to
  the devil," and Gen 4:7 "If you do what is
  right, will you not be accepted? But if you do
  not do what is right, sin is crouching at your
  door; it desires to have you, but you must
  rule over it."
- o So, while it may be true that personal sin may
  not cause every illness, Scripture shows that
  it can most certainly be the case. And the
  roots of sickness and disease are identified
  by Jesus as the work of the devil and not the
  Father because everywhere Jesus went He
  destroyed the work of sickness.
- o Moreover, Jesus later sent the twelve and the
  seventy-two to heal the sick and cast out
  devils wherever they found them. Jesus, the
  Son of God, became "fashioned as a man"
  (Phi 2:8), put on human flesh, and healed the

sick by faith through the power of God. He gave that same healing power to the twelve apostles and later the seventy-two. These men also healed the sick by faith. That same healing power is available for us, by faith today, to destroy the work of sickness and disease in our own bodies and wherever we encounter it.

o If it were God's plan to just rain down healing from Heaven, why would He use men and women on earth in the Old and New Testament (including Jesus) to minister healing individually?

o God's equation, His will, and His plan for healing are His power and grace, plus our faith and, in some cases, our obedience to depart from sin. Many times, Jesus asked a person to take a faith action or step and/or asked, "Do you believe I am able to do this?" (see Mat 9:28, Mar 5:36, Mar 9:23, Mar 11:23-24, Luk 8:50)

o I have to insert here that often, when people who don't believe in healing talk about God humbling someone or sending them sickness to teach them a lesson, it includes people who don't recover. The man born blind was healed. Saul, who was blinded and became Paul, was healed.

- *It is always God's will to heal a person physically. Paul's testimony teaches the contrary, that is it not always God's will to heal us in this life* (2 Corinthians 12:7–10).

- o 2 Cor 12:7–10 (ESV): "So to keep me from becoming conceited because of the surpassing greatness of the revelations, a thorn was given me in the flesh, a messenger of Satan to harass me, to keep me from becoming conceited. Three times I pleaded with the Lord about this, that it should leave me. But he said to me "My grace is sufficient for you, for my power is made perf ect in weakness." Therefore, I will boast all the more gladly of my weaknesses, so that the power of Christ may rest upon me. For the sake of Christ, then, I am content with weaknesses, insults, hardships, persecutions, and calamities. For when I am weak, then I am strong."
- o I have written a chapter on "Paul's thorn in the flesh" in "The Bible Promises of Healing Vol I." In short, I believe the Bible shows that the "messenger" that was given by "Satan to harass" Paul was a demon.
- o Easton's Bible Dictionary Messenger: (Hebrew mal'ak, Greek angelos), an angel, a messenger who runs on foot, the bearer of dispatches.
- o Satan led a third of the angels in rebellion against God. When they lost, they were cast

into the earth. The Bible refers to them as demons.

- o I believe this "thorn," this angel "given" by Satan, went about harassing and persecuting Paul by stirring up mobs to beat him, stone him, imprison him, cause shipwrecks, etc., to stop him from sharing the revelation of the risen Christ. I believe the devil similarly inspired Herod to put Peter in prison.
- o The devil also stirred up mobs against Jesus to try to stop the flow of revelation that Jesus was indeed the Christ, the son of the living God.
- o I believe God could not take away the persecutions and mobs, even after Paul prayed three times, because God has not promised to take the devil and his demons away until Jesus' return. Until that time, we are told to rely on His grace or, as He told Paul, "My grace is sufficient for thee."
- o There is Bible evidence that the devil has come against every powerful messenger who has carried the revelation of God's mercy, love, forgiveness, goodness, salvation, healing, grace, and power.
- o I believe he inspired the killing of the Old Testament prophets. He was behind Ahab's chasing of Elijah with an army and raising up Jezebel to paralyze him with fear and go into hiding. He inspired Pharaoh to kill all the

newborn baby boys to prevent the exaltation of Moses and inspired similar killings to prevent the arrival of Jesus. The devil inspired persecution against Daniel and got him thrown in the lion's den. He got the three Hebrew boys thrown into the fire. The devil inspired Haman to go after Esther and later to try to get all the Jews killed. And I believe he inspired Heord's daughter to ask for the head of John the Baptist.

o Satan came himself to try to deceive Jesus in the wilderness. When deception didn't work, Satan brought full-scale persecution against Jesus. The devil's work is to snuff out the light of the glorious gospel of Christ, the revelation of God the Son. Satan did not want the revelation of Jesus, the Word of God, to be exalted in the earth, especially after Jesus' death. The thorn was "Satan's messenger," not God at work trying to keep Paul from being exalted or proud.

o I ask this of those who would still cling to the notion that the same God who gives an "abundance of revelation" (as was given to Paul) punishes those with sickness and disease for receiving the revelations. Where are your revelations? Where are the revelations that were given to you that were so powerful that you had to be humbled by God? It doesn't make sense.

- o Only the devil stands to gain by blocking
    revelation from God. The devil is the one
    who stirred up people to kill the prophets in
    the Old Testament and to kill Jesus and Paul
    in the New Testament.
  - o God does not reveal His Word or release
    revelation and then try to thwart or hinder it
    by sending sickness and disease to the
    person He gave the revelation.
- *If a person is not healed, the blame lies in that person's lack of faith. This overlooks the fact that Jesus once healed a man who had no faith at all (John 5:1–9).*
  - o "Jhn 5:1–9 (ESV): "After this there was a feast
    of the Jews, and Jesus went up to Jerusalem.
    Now there is in Jerusalem by the Sheep Gate
    a pool, in Aramaic called Bethesda, which has
    five roofed colonnades. In these lay a
    multitude of invalids—blind, lame, and
    paralyzed. One man was there who had been
    an invalid for thirty-eight years. When Jesus
    saw him lying there and knew that he had
    already been there a long time, he said to
    him, 'Do you want to be healed?' The sick
    man answered him, 'Sir, I have no one to put
    me into the pool when the water is stirred
    up, and while I am going another steps down
    before me.' Jesus said to him, 'Get up, take
    up your bed, and walk.' And at once the man

was healed, and he took up his bed and walked."

- o The writer of the commentary totally missed it here. Yes, the man's initial response seems to indicate that he has no faith in being healed because he believes that he can't get to the healing pool when it is stirred. However, when Jesus tells him to take up his bed and walk, the man takes a faith step and tries to get up even though he has been lame for 38 years!
- o What an incredible act of faith that was! The Bible says that "faith without works is dead" (Jam 2:14-26). The commentary writer missed that Jesus often asked the person needing healing to take a faith step or action as a demonstration of their faith.
- o In Matthew chapter 12, Jesus tells a man with a withered hand to "Stretch forth thine hand. And he stretched it forth; and it was restored whole, like as the other."
- o In John Chapter 9, Jesus tells a man born blind to go wash after he had put mud on his eyes (Jhn 9:6-7): "Having said these things, he spit on the ground and made mud with the saliva. Then he anointed the man's eyes with the mud and said to him, 'Go, wash in the pool of Siloam' (which means Sent). So he went and washed and came back seeing."

o In Luke chapter 17, we see Jesus tell ten lepers to take a faith step to receive their healing. Luk 17:12-14: "Then as He entered a certain village, there met Him ten men who were lepers, who stood afar off. And they lifted up their voices and said, 'Jesus, Master, have mercy on us!' So when He saw them, He said to them, 'Go, show yourselves to the priests.' And so it was that as they went, they were cleansed."

o In this case, it wasn't enough for the ten lepers to verbally express their belief that Jesus could heal them by asking for mercy. Jesus required them to take a faith step. He told the leper in Mat 8:3 to take a similar step.

o According to a commentary I found on Mat 8:3, this was a big step of faith in that it required them to go against the existing laws governing lepers: "The leper in the story acted contrary to the instructions, stipulated in Leviticus 13-14, of how persons with such skin diseases should act. Being contagious and unclean persons, lepers were supposed to isolate themselves from others, demonstrate their impurity and warn people of their illness." (Society, n.d.)

In Acts chapter 3, Peter follows the same pattern as Jesus when he heals a man lame from his mother's womb, Act 3:6-8: "Then Peter said, silver and gold have I none; but such as I have give I thee: In the name of Jesus Christ of Nazareth rise up and walk. And he took him by the right hand, and lifted him up: and immediately his feet and ankle bones received strength. And he leaping up stood, and walked, and entered with them into the temple, walking, and leaping, and praising God."

People like the author of the commentary above don't understand that modern-day workers of miracles and those operating with healing gifts are copying a biblical pattern. How is Jesus saying, "Get up, take up your bed, and walk" in Jhn 5:8 or Peter saying it in Acts 3:6 different from a "faith healer" telling someone to get out of a wheelchair?

The author of the commentary doesn't understand what's happening in modern times because they don't understand the pattern of Scripture. This pattern extends back to the Old Testament. In 2 Kings chapter 5, Naaman was told by the prophet Elisha to go "wash himself" seven times in the Jordan River to be healed of leprosy.

Until Naaman took this faith step, he couldn't be healed. God sent a means of healing through the prophet Elisha, but Naaman had to respond in faith, take the faith step of washing in the dirty Jordan River, to receive the healing that God had already made available.

"And He was casting out a demon, and it was mute. So it was, when the demon had gone out, that the mute spoke; and the multitudes marveled. But some of them said, "He casts out demons by Beelzebub, the ruler of the demons." Others, testing Him, sought from Him a sign from heaven. But He, knowing their thoughts, said to them: "Every kingdom divided against itself is brought to desolation, and a house divided against a house falls. If Satan also is divided against himself, how will his kingdom stand? Because you say I cast out demons by Beelzebub. And if I cast out demons by Beelzebub, by whom do your sons cast them out? Therefore they will be your judges. But if I cast out demons with the finger of God, surely the kingdom of God has come upon you. When a strong man, fully armed, guards his own palace, his goods are in peace. But when a stronger than he comes upon him and overcomes him, he takes from him all his armor in which he trusted, and divides his spoils. He who is not with Me is against Me, and he who does not gather with Me scatters."

If the greatest healing evangelists of my grandmother's generation were false teachers, healed the sick, and cast out devils, isn't that a house divided against itself? Or is it more likely that the writers of this commentary are more like those who sought to test Jesus and call him a false teacher?

Where is it written anywhere in Scripture that God has stopped giving the Eph 4 and 1 Cor 12 gifts of apostle, prophet, evangelist, teacher, pastor, miracle worker, those with gifts of healing, administrators, helpers, and those who interpret tongues?

None of these writers would say that God has stopped setting the gifts of the Church's pastors, teachers, administrators, and helpers. Their own lack of knowledge, understanding, and faith has caused them to say without any Scriptural evidence that God stopped setting certain gifts in the Church.

Writers of the commentary I presented want us to stop pursuing God's exhortation to "earnestly covet or desire the best gifts":

"And God hath set some in the church, first apostles, secondarily prophets, thirdly teachers, after that miracles, then gifts of healings, helps, governments, diversities of tongues. Are all apostles? Are all prophets? Are all teachers? Are all workers of miracles? Have all the gifts of healing? Do all speak with tongues? Do all interpret? But covet earnestly the best gifts: and yet shew I unto you a more excellent way."

1 Cor 12:28-31 (KJV)

"Now concerning spiritual gifts, brethren, I would not have you ignorant. Ye know that ye were Gentiles, carried away unto these dumb idols, even as ye were led. Wherefore I give you to understand, that no man speaking by the Spirit of God calleth Jesus accursed: and that no man can say that Jesus is the Lord, but by the Holy Ghost. Now there are diversities of gifts, but the same Spirit. And there are differences of administrations, but the same Lord. And there are diversities of operations, but it is the same God which worketh all in all. But the manifestation of the Spirit is given to every man to profit withal. For to one is given by the Spirit the word of wisdom; to another the word of knowledge by the same Spirit; To another faith by the same Spirit; to another the gifts of healing by the same Spirit; To another the working of miracles; to another prophecy; to another discerning of spirits; to another divers kinds of tongues; to another the interpretation of tongues: But all these worketh that one and the selfsame Spirit, dividing to every man severally as he will."

1 Cor 12:1-11

The Bible says in 1 Corinthians chapter 12 that there are spiritual "gifts," "diversities of gifts," and differences in "administrations" and "operations" of those gifts. It further says that God, through the Holy Spirit, is "working" through the manifestation of those gifts. In 1 Cor 12:31, the Bible urges us to "covet" or desire "earnestly the best gifts." So, being a miracle worker or someone who operates with gifts of healing is something the Bible says I should covet.

The Bible says I could desire these gifts and pray that the Holy Spirit, as He chooses, would work those through me. I can desire and ask God that by the Holy Spirit, I could begin to work miracles and operate with healing gifts. That was an amazing revelation to me!

Paul said he was "called to be an Apostle," "set apart for the gospel" (Rom 1:1, 1 Cor 1:1). We know that Paul responded in faith to his call and began operating as an apostle. Is it possible that those who sense that they are called to be workers of miracles and operate with gifts of healing become "set" in the body of Christ as they respond in faith according to 1 Cor 12:28?

The Holy Spirit has not stopped operating, so the gifts are still available to those who earnestly covet them. We all have different gifts that operate by faith by the will, grace, and power of the Holy Ghost.

"For I say, through the grace given unto me, to every man that is among you, not to think of himself more highly than he ought to think; but to think soberly, according as God hath dealt to every man the measure of faith. For as we have many members in one body, and all members have not the same office: So we, being many, are one body in Christ, and every one members one of another. Having then gifts differing according to the grace that is given to us, whether prophecy, let us prophesy according to the proportion of faith; Or ministry, let us wait on our ministering: or he that teacheth, on teaching; Or he that exhorteth, on exhortation: he that giveth, let him do it with simplicity; he that ruleth, with diligence; he that sheweth mercy, with cheerfulness."

"There are diversities of gifts, but the same Spirit. There are differences of ministries, but the same Lord. And there are diversities of activities, but it is the same God who works all in all. But the manifestation of the Spirit is given to each one for the profit of all: for to one is given the word of wisdom through the Spirit, to another the word of knowledge through the same Spirit, to another faith by the same Spirit, to another gifts of healings by the same Spirit, to another the working of miracles, to another prophecy, to another discerning of spirits, to another different kinds of tongues, to another the interpretation of tongues. But one and the same Spirit works all these things, distributing to each one individually as He wills. For as the body is one and has many members, but all the members of that one body, being many, are one body, so also is Christ. For by one Spirit we were all baptized into one body—whether Jews or Greeks, whether slaves or free—and have all been made to drink into one Spirit. For in fact the body is not one member but many. If the foot should say, 'Because I am not a hand, I am not of the body,' is it therefore not of the

body? And if the ear should say, 'Because I am
not an eye, I am not of the body,' is it therefore
not of the body? If the whole body were an eye,
where would be the hearing? If the
whole were hearing, where would be the
smelling? But now God has set the members,
each one of them, in the body just as He
pleased. And if they were all one member,
where would the body be? But now
indeed there are many members, yet one
body. And the eye cannot say to the hand, 'I
have no need of you'; nor again the head to the
feet, 'I have no need of you.' No, much rather,
those members of the body which seem to be
weaker are necessary. And those members of
the body which we think to be less honorable,
on these we bestow greater honor; and our
unpresentable parts have greater modesty, but
our presentable parts have no need. But God
composed the body, having given greater honor
to that part which lacks it, that there should be
no schism in the body, but that the members
should have the same care for one another. And
if one member suffers, all the members suffer
with it; or if one member is honored, all the
members rejoice with it."

1 Cor 12:4-26

I think it is fascinating and significant that God placed the "can the eye say to the hand, I have no need of you" analogy in the middle of His discussion of spiritual gifts, gifts that include working of miracles and healings. No one church has all the revelations. I went to a church that had great revelation on faith, healing, and prosperity but frowned upon psychology and even the use of Christian therapists.

Currently, I go to a church that doesn't believe in healing or prosperity. Still, they believe in the love of God and areas of emotional healing that I've never seen anywhere else. This church also greatly emphasizes the type of compassion Jesus ministered to the woman at the well, the woman caught in adultery, and the harlot who washed Jesus' feet. I haven't seen this in very many places in the body of Christ. And so, I go there for that, and I go there for the fellowship. But I would not trust my life on what they say about healing, and I've seen too much in my own life in terms of blessings to listen to anything they say about prosperity.

I recently found a quote by noted theologian A. W. Tozer that let me know that my situation was not unique or even new, for that matter:

"How many blessed truths have you gotten snowed under. People believe them, but they are just not being taught, that is all. Here was a man and his wife, a very fine intelligent couple from another city. They named the church to which they belonged, and I instantly said, 'That is a fine church!'

'Oh, yes,' they said, 'but they don't teach what we came over here for.' They came over because they were ill and wanted to be scripturally anointed for healing. So I got together two missionaries, two preachers and an elder, and we anointed them and prayed for them. If you were to go to that church where they attended and say to the preacher, 'Do you believe that the Lord answers prayer and heals the sick?' He would reply, 'Sure I do!' He believes it, but he doesn't teach it, and what you don't believe strongly enough to teach doesn't do you any good."

A.W. Tozer "How to Be Filled with the Holy Spirit, pg 12 Moody Publishers 2016

The Holy Spirit still manifests all His gifts through men and women today. We can't say that we do not need this gift or that gift. We certainly can't choose to say that the Holy Spirit has ceased operating in certain gifts because we don't think they are needed today or because someone has faked the operation of the gifts.

There is always an imitation or fake where there is a genuine article. When Moses' staff turned into a snake, Pharoah's magicians were able to imitate the miracle (Exo 7:11-13). Certainly, there have been men and women who have not been called into any office and have tried to imitate genuine moves of the Holy Spirit just as the sons of Sceva tried to imitate the casting out of devils (Act 19:11-20).

I had a Pastor named George Thompson, a millionaire who said, "I don't take financial advice from broke folks." Though humorous, I still abide by that today. Similarly, I don't receive "spiritual advice" related to healing from those who don't have a revelation of healing and miracles.

One of my favorite Bible teachers, Keith Moore, said, "We teach healing, and we see healings." He said this in response to another pastor who asked why he didn't see healings manifested in his church. That pastor, like the one in the A. W. Tozer quote, believed healings were possible but didn't believe it enough to teach it in his church. Rom 10:17 (NKJV) says, "So then faith comes by hearing, and hearing by the word of God."

If we want to see the Holy Spirit manifest the gifts of healing and working miracles, we must go to a place where the Word of God is being preached about the operation of these gifts versus where they say we have no need of them today.

We need to hear the Word of God on healing and miracles to add our faith to it, mix our faith with it so that it will prosper (Isa 55:11), and benefit us.

"For unto us was the gospel preached, as well as unto them: but the word preached did not profit them, not being mixed with faith in them that heard it."

Heb 4:2

I conclude this chapter with biographical snippets of some of the greatest healing evangelists. You can research the lives of these great men and women and see that they espoused the same Scriptural principles that were modeled for us by Jesus, the twelve apostles, and Paul.

Smith Wigglesworth, for example, practiced fasting before dealing with the sick. He believed it was necessary for those whose sickness was demonically inspired. Smith Wigglesworth followed the example of Jesus in Scripture and received the same result. Jesus healed the boy the disciples could not heal, who was deaf and dumb and kept being thrown into the fire and water. First, he rebuked them for their lack of faith, then said, "This kind cometh not out but by prayer and fasting." This kind of what? This kind of demonic spirit.

Smith Wigglesworth

"However, Wigglesworth's real calling card was something that's all but lost in the modern Pentacostal faith: healing." (Shilling, 2016)

"Smith would pray and the blind would see, and the deaf were healed, people came out of wheelchairs, and cancers were destroyed. One remarkable story is when He prayed for a woman in a hospital. While he and a friend were praying she died. He took her out of the bed stood her against the wall and said 'in the name of Jesus I rebuke this death'. Her whole body began to tremble. The he said 'in the name of Jesus walk', and she walked. Everywhere he would go he would teach and then show the power of God. He began to receive requests from all over the world. He taught in Europe, Asia, New Zealand and many other areas. When the crowds became very large he began a 'wholesale healing'. He would have everyone who needed healing lay hands on themselves and then he would pray. Hundreds would be healed at one time.

Over Smith's ministry it was confirmed that 14 people were raised from the dead. Thousands were saved and healed and he impacted whole continents for Christ." (Healing and Revival.com, n.d.)

Oral Roberts

"From Poverty to America's Healing Evangelist

Oral Roberts is one of the best known healing evangelists of the 20th Century... During a sociology class at Phillips University in Enid, he heard God speak: 'Son, don't be like other men. Don't be like any denomination. Be like Jesus and heal like he did.' From that moment, Roberts determined that he would take God's message of healing to his generation. He moved his family to Tulsa and began to hold crusades across the US.

From 1947-1962, Oral Roberts' large scale tent crusades changed the religious landscape of American evangelicalism. Oral Roberts' name became synonymous with healing. Across the

United States, millions of people came to his large tent crusades to hear his dynamic preaching and to witness first hand the power of God as he prayed with people. Millions of people came to Christ and were healed in his ministry.... Oral Robers University (ORU) was founded as a different kind of Christian University... ORU drew students from a variety of theological backgrounds, all unified by a belief in the Holy Spirit and healing. This was demonstrated in 1968 when he joined the Methodist Church in order to expand the ecumenical reach of his ministry. Although the move was ultimately detrimental to Roberts' Pentecostal support base, he believed it fulfilled God's call to bring healing power to his generation."

(Isgrigg, 2021)

William Branham

"The American prophet and evangelist William Branham was, for all intents and purposes, another such man. Initiator of the post-war healing revival. Branham claimed that throughout his later life he was guided by an angel who first appeared to him in a secret cave in 1946. Preaching to congregations of thousands (sometimes 20,000 would attend his meetings), his ministry was characterised by amazing manifestations of healing and the word of knowledge. Church historian David Harrell says of him: 'The power of a Branham service... remains a legend unparalleled in the history of the charismatic movement.'... The American evangelist, TL Osborn, told of his visit to a Branham healing meeting: 'I was especially captivated by the deliverance of a little deaf-mute girl over whom he prayed thus: 'Thou deaf and dumb spirit, I adjure thee in Jesus' name, leave the child.' When he snapped his fingers, the girl heard and spoke perfectly.'

Very often, as people approached him in the healing line, Branham would describe their illness, other unknown information about them, and sometimes even call them by name. The gift, many people insisted, was 100 percent accurate. Walter J Hollenweger, who interpreted for Branham in Zurich, said that he was 'not aware of any case in which he was mistaken in the often detailed statements he made'.

The Canadian charismatic leader, Ern Baxter, who knew Branham well and worked extensively with him for seven years, also testified to the tremendous accuracy of his words of knowledge:

'Before praying for a person, he would give accurate details concerning the person's ailments, and also details of their lives – their home town, activities, actions – even way back in their childhood. Branham never once made a mistake with the word of knowledge in all the years I was with him. That covers, in my case, thousands of instances.'" (Publishing, n.d.)

A. A. Allen

"He left the pastorate and began to hold meetings as a singing healing evangelist. In Missouri a coal miner who had been blind for several years was healed. Allen held meetings and was constantly on the road. This was a strain for Lexie and their four children. Income was not stable and the responsibility was wearing on her. In 1947 Allen accepted a call to pastor a church in Corpus Christi, Texas. He wanted to settle down and have a family life. The church blossomed. Allen had a vision for reaching more people. He wanted to start a radio ministry. The church turned him down and he was devastated. He realized, over time, the enemy had taken advantage of his hurt and attacked him

In 1949 the healing revival, notably led
by William Branham, was making news. He was
incredulous at first, but felt stirred to look into
what was happening. He went to an Oral Roberts
tent revival meeting. He realized as he watched
what was happening that this was the ministry
God had called him to. He had been unwilling to
pay the price to see it, however. He resigned
his pastorate, in 1950, and once again began
holding evangelistic meetings. People would be
healed in their seats as he preached. He also had
his first article in the influential 'Voice of Healing'
magazine put out by Gordon Lindsay." (Healing
and Revival.com, n.d.)

T. L. Osborn

"God wasn't finished with the Osborns yet. He
had heard their cries to see and hear the reality
that Jesus still did miracles. In September 1947
the couple returned to pastor Montaville
Tabernacle in Portland, Oregon. William
Branhan was traveling with Jack
Moore and Gordon Lindsay holding healing
meetings. They held meetings in November 1947
at the Portland Civic Auditorium. Daisy attended
a meeting first because T. L. was in the midst of
a denominational convention. She told T. L.

about the meetings and he knew he had to attend. The healings and miracles in Branham's meetings were dramatic. He would call people out by name, tell them their sicknesses, and then pray for them and they would be healed. The Osborns were overwhelmed with a new vision of the love of Jesus and the fact that He is the same 'yesterday, today, and forever.' What impressed T. L. the most was that Branham exalted Jesus and showed Jesus' ability to love and heal people. He saw Branham as a humble man simply doing what Jesus asked him to do. T. L. began weeping at what he saw Jesus doing. The blind saw, the deaf heard, and the crippled walked. T. L. said it was as if he heard a thousand voices saying 'you can do that too.' Once more the couple was shaken to their roots.

The Osborns decided to read the Bible in a new way. They read about the miracles and the fact that Jesus gave His disciples the authority to do what He did. T. L. fasted all food and water for three days as he sought God's presence. The Lord spoke to him and said 'As I've been with others, so I will be with you. Wherever you go, I will give you the land for your possession. No demon, no disease, or no power can stand before you all the days of your life, IF you get the people to believe my Word.' They began to hold healing meetings at their church. Immediately they began to see healings and miracles. Their first miracle was a woman who had been badly injured in a car accident and could barely walk with crutches. She came under the power of God and started walking normally around the room with her eyes closed. When she opened her eyes she was completely healed and gave testimony that she had heard an angelic choir singing the praises of God.

The missionary flame in the Osborns rose up once again. Now that they were seeing healings and miracles they felt they had the answer to reach the lost in foreign lands. They didn't have a lot of money but they were invited to go to Jamaica and preach in early 1949. They became affiliated with the Voice of Healing Organization. They returned to the US and held meetings with William Branham, F. F. Bosworth, and Gordon Lindsay. These meetings gave T. L. national attention, but the Osborns hearts were for the lost in foreign lands. Between 1950 and 1964 the couple held large crusades in 40 countries. In 1953 the Osborns formed the Association of Native Evangelism made up of local pastors to plant churches. The meetings were some of the largest ever held before that time. The meetings would often have tens of thousands of people attending, with large numbers of people being saved. Wherever they went their ministry was marked by dramatic miracles and healings."

(Healing and Revival.com, n.d.)

Kathryn Kuhlman

"Kathryn Johanna Kuhlman was born on May 9, 1907, in Concordia, Missouri. Her parents were German and she was one of four children. Her mother was a harsh disciplinarian, who showed little love or affection. On the other hand, she had an extremely close and loving relationship with her father. She would describe, as a small child how, her father would come home from work and she would hang on his leg and cling to him. She often said that her relationship with God the Father was extremely real because of her relationship with her own father.

Kuhlman was converted when she was 14 at an evangelistic meeting held in a small Methodist church. When she was 16 she graduated from high school, which only went to tenth grade in their town. He older sister Myrtle had married an Itinerant evangelist, Everett B. Parrott. They spent their time traveling and asked that Kathryn could join them for the summer. Her parents agreed and she went to Oregon to help out. She worked with them, and often gave her testimony. When the summer was over she wanted to stay, and the couple agreed. She ended up working with them for five years.

The evangelistic team was made up of four people, Everette, Myrtle, Kathryn, and a pianist named Helen Gulliford. In 1928 Everette missed a meeting in Boise, Idaho. Myrtle and Kathryn preached to cover for Everette. The pastor of the church encouraged Kathryn to step out on her own. Helen agreed to join her. Her first sermon was in a run-down pool hall in Boise, Idaho. The team covered Idaho, Utah, and Colorado for the following five years. In 1933 they moved to Pueblo, Colorado. They set up in an abandoned Montgomery Ward warehouse. They stayed there for six months.

Denver, being a much bigger city, was the next stop. They moved several times but ended up in a paper company's warehouse, which they named the Kuhlman Revival Tabernacle. Then in 1935 they moved once more to an abandoned truck garage they named the Denver Revival Tabernacle. Kathryn was seeing a lot of success in Denver. The church grew to about 2000 members. She began a radio show called

'Smiling Through' and invited speakers from all over the country. One of them was Phil Kerr who taught on divine healing. In 1935 another invited evangelist was Burroughs Waltrip.

Waltrip was bad news for Kuhlman. He was a charismatic, handsome man several years older than she was. There was an immediate attraction, and one family claims to have seen the couple embracing in 1935, but he was married and had two children. Waltrip left Denver and went home to Austin, Texas, but the relationship simmered between Kuhlman and Waltrip. In 1937 he was invited back to Denver to take the pulpit for two months. Shortly after he divorced his wife and abandoned his two sons. He then spread the story that his wife had left him. He moved to Mason City, Iowa, where he told everyone he was single, and started a new ministry. Waltrip raised pledges of $70,000 to build a ministry building called Radio Chapel. It was state of the art with a disappearing pulpit and an art deco style. He appeared to be a successful and dynamic preacher.

There was an ongoing relationship between Kuhlman and Waltrip, and they married in September 1938. Kuhlman was naïve about the consequences of her choices and the marriage was a disaster. She announced to her church that she and Waltrip were married and they would go between Denver and Mason City preaching at their two churches. Most of the people in her congregation left due to her relationship with Waltrip. She gave up her church in Denver, lost some of her closest associates, and moved to Mason City. Waltrip's success turned out to be a pipe dream as well. The Radio Chapel was completed in June of 1938. By October 1938 Waltrip could not meet his debts. In December Waltrip was demanding a higher salary, even with the shortfall in income. His Board of Directors quit and left him to deal with the finances. His solution was not to pay the mortgage or debts on the Chapel. Radio Chapel went into bankruptcy. Waltrip's last sermon was in May 1939. The Waltrips were on their own. Kathryn's happy vision of she and her husband flying back and forth between Denver and Mason City with a successful preaching careers was utterly demolished.

The next few years were very hard for the couple. They embarked on the road as traveling evangelists, primarily staying in the Midwest. They were not accepted in many places due to their marriage history. Initial advertisements listed Waltrip as the primary evangelist. Then occasionally Mrs. Waltrip was also mentioned. By the early 1940s Kathryn Kuhlman Waltrip was given equal billing. Finally by the mid-1940s Kathryn was using only Kathryn Kuhlman in meetings where she was the primary speaker. In 1944 Kuhlman went on an evangelistic tour on the east coast without Waltrip. It may have been a conscious decision to leave him, or she may also have taken the opportunity to reassess her life. It appears to have been more gradual as Waltrip wrote about them as a couple as late as 1946. Kuhlman never returned to Waltrip and they eventually divorced in 1947. She left her marriage behind and from then on acted as if it never existed in the first place.

In 1946 Kuhlman was asked to speak in Franklin, Pennsylvania. She was well received and decided to stay in the area. Kuhlman began preaching on radio broadcasts in Oil City, Pennsylvania. These became so popular they were picked up in Pittsburgh, and she was preaching throughout the area. She began to preach about the healing power of God. In 1947 a woman was healed of a tumor while listening to Kuhlman preach. Several Sundays later a man was also healed while she was teaching on the Holy Spirit. She was now convinced of God's healing work. One important thing to note is the context and timing of this breakout period in Kuhlman's life. 1947 was the beginning of the Healing Revival (sometimes referred to as the Latter Rain Revival) that would last for the next 10 years. What was happening in Kuhlman's meetings was breaking out across the United States. It was in this time frame that the Voice of Healing Ministry was established and men like William Branham, Oral Roberts, A.A. Allen and many others were propelled onto the public stage. Kuhlman was not associated with those groups, but stepped into the flow of what God's Spirit was doing across the nation and the world.

In 1948 Kuhlman held a series of meetings at Carnegie Hall in Pittsburgh. She eventually moved to Pittsburgh in 1950 and continued to hold meetings at Carnegie Hall until 1971. She was used by God to bring the charismatic message to many denominational churches, including the Catholic Church. (She received a lot of criticism over this and was accused of being a closet Catholic.) These were her best known years. Her style was flamboyant. She would hold her famous miracle services and the auditorium was filled to capacity every time. She was on radio and television shows. She was ordained in 1968 by the Evangelical Church Alliance. Hundreds of people were healed in her meetings, and even while listening to her on the radio or television. People she prayed for would often be hit with the power of God and be 'slain in the Spirit.' Kuhlman never claimed that she was the healer. She always pointed people to Jesus as their healer.

Kuhlman had been diagnosed with a heart problem in 1955. She kept a very busy schedule and overworked herself, especially in the 1970's traveling back and forth from Pittsburgh to Los Angeles frequently, as well as taking trips around the world. Her heart was enlarged and Kuhlman died on February 20, 1976, in Tulsa, following open-heart surgery. Videos of some of her services are still available and continue to be popular today." (Healing and Revival.com, n.d.)

No PrIvate Interpretation

2 Pet 1:20-21"says, "Knowing this first, that no prophecy of the scripture is of any private interpretation. For the prophecy came not in old time by the will of man: but holy men of God spake as they were moved by the Holy Ghost." In this book, I will not share some personal revelation or interpretation. I will share Scripture upon Scripture that highlights God's promises and His will for healing.

All too often, I have witnessed that people, even pastors and preachers, take the Word of God and unknowingly bend it to match their personal experience. I believe, particularly in the area of healing, that for many people, their personal experience is so powerful, so overwhelming that it clouds their understanding and interpretation of the Scriptures on healing. They shrink the timeless revelation and inexhaustible power of the Word of the Almighty God in Heaven down to match their unique, fleeting experiences on Earth.

I attended a church years ago and was shocked to hear a well-known pastor say from the pulpit, "First God took my dad, now He took my momma!" He talked about how angry he was with God. This preacher had a seminary education and degrees, but his personal experience with healing shaped his doctrine on healing and was now influencing the beliefs of thousands.

Recently, in another church, I heard a pastor denounce prosperity preachers as false teachers. He started with the financial area of prosperity but then moved into the area of healing. 3 Jhn 2 (NKJV)"says, "Beloved, I pray that you may prosper in all things and be in health, just as your soul prospers." The pastor literally began to preach against the 3 John 2 promise of prosperity in our bodies.

He began to try to explain that God doesn't answer all of our prayers for healing, though he didn't know why. But unfortunately, he went further. He began to try to show in Scripture that for some people, the promises of God are not fulfilled.

I will walk through the specific Scriptures the pastor used in the next chapter, but I have to point out that he tied it to the death of a dear loved one. He said, "he'd done everything," and she still died. He said that it caused him to challenge his beliefs. I agonized over his loss, but all I could think of was how his loss might be affecting his theology and now influencing hundreds of others. I had my first hint of this bending of the Scriptures with this same pastor on a previous occasion.

The month prior, the pastor spoke of a child in Scripture with "epilepsy." He went on to share a very personal and engaging story about a seizure he had as a child. However, my spirit got stuck on the word epilepsy because I was sure that word wasn't in the Bible.

When he spoke of a boy with "epilepsy," I was sure he was talking about a Biblical account where a man's son kept being thrown into the fire and water in an attempt to kill him, and the apostles couldn't heal him.

In that passage of Scripture, Jesus rebuked the disciples for their lack of faith but added, "This kind cometh not out but by prayer and fasting." The pastor indeed was talking about the boy in Mark 9:14-29. Here's the account:

"And when He came to the disciples, He saw a great multitude around them, and scribes disputing with them. Immediately, when they saw Him, all the people were greatly amazed, and running to Him, greeted Him. And He asked the scribes, "What are you discussing with them?" Then one of the crowd answered and said, "Teacher, I brought You my son, who has <u>a mute spirit</u>. And wherever <u>it</u> seizes him, <u>it</u> throws him down; he foams at the mouth, gnashes his teeth, and becomes rigid. So I spoke to Your disciples, that they should cast it out, but

they could not." He answered him and said
"O faithless generation, how long shall I be with
you? How long shall I bear with you? Bring him
to Me." Then they brought him to Him.
And when he saw Him, immediately the <u>spirit</u>
convulsed him, and he fell on the ground and
wallowed, foaming at the mouth. So He asked
his father, "How long has this been happening to
him?" And he said, "From childhood. And often
<u>he</u> has thrown him both into the fire and into
the water to destroy him. But if You can do
anything, have compassion on us and help
us." Jesus said to him, "If you can believe, all
things are possible to him who believes."
Immediately the father of the child cried out and
said with tears, "Lord, I believe; help my
unbelief!" When Jesus saw that the people came
running together, He rebuked the <u>unclean spirit</u>,
saying to <u>it</u>, "Deaf and dumb <u>spirit</u>, I command
you, come out of him and enter him no
more!" Then the <u>spirit</u> cried out, convulsed him
greatly, and came out of him. And he became as
one dead, so that many said, "He is dead." But
Jesus took him by the hand and lifted him up,
and he arose. And when He had come into the
house, His disciples asked Him privately, "Why
could we not cast <u>it</u> out?" So He said to

them, "This <u>kind</u> can come out by nothing but prayer and fasting."

*underlining added for emphasis

As you can see with the underlining, over and over in the passage of Scripture, the cause of the boy's falls is identified as a "spirit." In Dr. Mike Freeman's Bible college, I was taught to look up the Hebrew and Greek meanings of words in the Old and New Testaments to see how their English translations affected their meaning.

The Greek word pneuma is translated as spirit in this passage. According to Strong's Greek concordance, it refers to "demons, or evil spirits, who were conceived as inhabiting the bodies of men." The Greek word akathartos, translated as "unclean" in the phrase "unclean spirit," means foul. So, the phrase could be read as "foul spirit." I also looked up the Greek words that described the spirit "crying out" and "convulsing" the boy. See Greek definitions below.

pneuma Strong's G4151 (spirit)

The KJV translates'Strong's G4151 in the following manner: Spirit (111x), Holy Ghost (89x), Spirit (of God) (13x), Spirit (of the Lord) (5x), (My) Spirit (3x), Spirit (of

truth) (3x), Spirit (of Christ) (2x), human
(spirit) (49x), (evil) spirit (47x), spirit
(general) (26x), spirit (8x), (Jesus' own) (6x),
'(Jesus' own) ghost (2x), miscellaneous (21x).

(Blue Letter Bible, n.d.)

akathartos (foul)
(Blue Letter Bible, n.d.)

krazō krad'-zo; a primary verb; properly, to
"croak" (as a raven) or scream, i.e. (genitive
case) to call aloud (shriek, exclaim, intreat):—cry
(out). (Blue Letter Bible, n.d.)

sparassō to convulse, tear
(Blue Letter Bible, n.d.)

In my efforts to search for epilepsy in the Bible, I
did find that the word or condition is mentioned in the
Bible (please see notes at the end of the chapter), but it
wasn't what the boy was experiencing in this passage of
Scripture.

We know from many examples in the Bible that
Jesus laid hands on the sick and healed them, and he

cast out demons, often by commanding them to come out. In this passage, we see Jesus commanding a "deaf and dumb spirit" to come out of the boy.

What then would cause this pastor to call the cause of this boy's condition epilepsy with the same conviction as if it were the written Word of God? What would cause him to replace the words of Jesus Himself with his own interpretation?

I don't know if the pastor found that the condition of epilepsy was mentioned in the Bible and mistakenly assumed that was what was happening in the passage or not. I also don't know if his personal experience affected his interpretation. I don't believe that the pastor intended to deceive. He is a man of incredible sincerity and a tremendous love for God. It is his most compelling quality.

However, this example highlights the importance of researching Scripture for ourselves. I have such a high regard for this pastor that I wasn't going to research what he said. But I believe the Holy Spirit prompted me to. It was the genesis of this entire book.

I have always been motivated to study the Scriptural support of those who don't believe in the healing principles of the Bible as I understand them.

"Making the word of God of none effect through your tradition, which ye have delivered: and many such like things do ye."

Mar 7:13

Again, I don't know if this pastor's experiences and "traditions" related to healing influenced his interpretation of the boy's account in Mark chapter 9. I do know, however, that with great sincerity and conviction, he mistakenly conveyed that what was happening to the boy was the illness epilepsy vs. what Jesus called a "deaf and dumb spirit.".

If Jesus' disciples could not heal the boy without the proper spiritual approach, how can we? If our religious traditions exclude the existence and operation of demons, could we ever expect to see healings of this kind? Was this interpretation important? Did the pastor's misinterpretation matter? It mattered to the father whose child was thrown into the fire and water. And I believe it could matter if we encountered something similar and wondered what the appropriate Scriptural remedy was.

*My research on the word epilepsy in the Bible

"An account of a boy with epileptic-like seizures is recorded in three of the four Gospels (Matthew 17:14–18; Mark 9:14–29; Luke 9:38–42). Only in Matthew's account (in the ESV and NKJV) is the word epileptic used to describe the boy; the NASB and KJV say 'lunatic,' based on the original Greek word's meaning of 'moonstruck.' The NIV says, 'He has seizures.' In Mark and Luke, the father of the boy states that his son is 'possessed by a spirit' and 'a spirit seizes him.' Comparing the three accounts in the Gospels, the boy's symptoms included sudden screaming, foaming at the mouth, lack of speech, falling, rigidity, and self-harm.

Matthew 17:14–18 says, 'When they came to the crowd, a man came up to him and, kneeling before him, said, 'Lord, have mercy on my son, for he is an epileptic and he suffers terribly. For often he falls into the fire, and often into the water. And I brought him to your disciples, and they could not heal him.' And Jesus answered, 'O faithless and twisted generation, how long am I to be with you? How long am I to bear with you? Bring him here to me.' And Jesus rebuked the demon, and it came out of him, and the boy was healed instantly' (ESV).

It is important to note that epilepsy was the father's assessment of his son's situation. Jesus, Matthew, Mark, and Luke all call it a demon, and Jesus cast it out as He did other demons. The seeming discrepancy in the three biblical accounts is probably due to the fact that the father said a lot of things in trying to get Jesus' attention. He was distraught, desperate for help, and at a loss to describe what was happening to his son. The fact that the father speaks of epilepsy in Matthew's account and calls it a 'spirit' in the other two Gospels does not create an irreconcilable difference. The father could easily have said all of the above as he described his son's condition. He did not know what was wrong. He only knew that he needed help.

The term epileptic is used only twice in the New Testament, in Matthew 17:15 and Matthew 4:24. The word translated 'epileptic' comes from the Greek word for 'lunatic.' In those days, the term could be applied to any type of seizures or behavior that resembled insanity. In New Testament times, people had no way to differentiate between brain disorders and demonic possession. Little was known about the causes or treatment of epilepsy, traumatic brain injury, or dementia, so it is understandable that the father in Matthew 17 would describe his son's behavior as epilepsy. But we know from Jesus' treatment of this boy that the child was in fact demon possessed (Mark 9:26).

However, the Bible does mention epilepsy as a condition separate from demon possession. Matthew 4:24 says, 'So his fame spread throughout all Syria, and they brought him all the sick, those afflicted with various diseases and pains, those oppressed by demons, epileptics, and paralytics, and he healed them' (emphasis added). Here epilepsy is listed with other physical ailments, indicating that epilepsy is a medical condition that can cause symptoms similar to demonic possession. Jesus healed epileptics, and He also cast out demons. The two conditions were not synonymous.

Although many inexplicable behaviors that affect the personality can be attributed to demonic oppression, we should never rush to judgment. Demons are still active and can possess and oppress people. Prayer and spiritual warfare can enable us to help those who are oppressed (2 Corinthians 10:4; Ephesians 6:12–17). But brain abnormalities or injury can also affect human behavior and can respond to medical treatment. Jesus always treated the individual, and He rarely healed the same disease in the same way. This shows us that we should also respond to individuals with sensitivity and discernment, using everything at our disposal to help and heal any way we can." (Got Questions, n.d.)

The "Unfulfilled" Promise

"These all died in faith, <u>not having received
the promises</u>, <u>but having seen them afar
off were assured of them</u>,
embraced them and confessed that they were
strangers and pilgrims on the earth...

And all these, having obtained a good testimony
through faith, <u>did not receive the promise</u>, <u>God
having provided something better for us</u>, that
they should not be made perfect apart from us."

*underlining added for emphasis

Heb 11:13, 39-40

"For I ell you, that many prophets and kings have
desired to see those things which you see,
and have not seen them; and to hear those
things which ye hear, and have not heard them."

Luk 10:24

"Concerning this salvation, the prophets, who
spoke of the grace that was to come to you,
searched intently and with the greatest

care, trying to find out the time and circumstances to which the Spirit of Christ in them was pointing when he predicted the sufferings of the Messiah and the glories that would follow. It was revealed to them that they were not serving themselves but you, when they spoke of the things that have now been told you by those who have preached the gospel to you by the Holy Spirit sent from heaven. Even angels long to look into these things."

1 Pet 1:10-12 (NIV)

In the previous chapter, I mentioned that I was at a church where the pastor took verses from Hebrews chapter 11 and tied them to the premise that God doesn't answer the promise of healing for all. He further emphasized that in this chapter, where so many great examples of faith are recorded, God highlighted examples where people didn't receive what God had promised.

The implication was that some people receive God's promise of healing while others don't. This was supposed to be an encouragement that even if we don't understand why God doesn't fulfill His promise to heal, we should still trust His goodness and sovereignty.

I have heard variants of this in other churches, and it sounded like this, "God is mysterious, and we don't always understand what He does," or "God's ways are higher than our ways, and we don't always understand why some prayers aren't answered," etc.

Someday, I will unpack that in an entire book. For now, let's go back and address the premise that God specifically put verses 13, 39, and 40 in the book of Hebrews to let us know that He doesn't always answer His "promises" for healing.

First, I find it interesting that in this line of reasoning, healing is understood as something "promised" by God. Therefore, those who follow this line of reasoning must know that some Scriptures "promise" healing to the believer.

I know that this pastor believes that God is honest and can't lie and that He is good and wants us to have good things. How does he reconcile God not fulfilling His "promise" of healing? How do others who believe like him explain it? The answer? They refer to Scriptures like this to explain why God didn't answer His healing "promise."

The underlying rationale is that God is not a liar or evil; we just don't fully understand Scripture. Further, through more Scripture study, we would understand that healing is not "promised" to all.

2 Tim 2:15 says, "Study to shew thyself approved unto God, a workman that needeth not to be ashamed, rightly dividing the word of truth." Act 17:11 (NIV) says, "Now the Berean Jews were of more noble character than those in Thessalonica, for they received the message with great eagerness and examined the Scriptures every day to see if what Paul said was true." As believers, we have an obligation to God to study the Scriptures.

We are not relieved of that obligation because the pastor or teacher is a sincere man of God (as this pastor is), a great orator, operates in the gifts of the Spirit, has multiple seminary degrees, etc. The Bible commends the Bereans for examining what Paul taught. And Paul was the writer of most of the New Testament and arguably the greatest apostle of all!

I'm not saying take a critical or judgemental stance against everything a pastor or teacher says. I am saying that it is our responsibility before God to examine the Word that is sown into our hearts. The verses this pastor quoted from Hebrews are the Word of God. But he was incorrect in his interpretation that the unfulfilled promise in these verses pertained to healing.

Jhn 14:26 (NKJV), Jesus says, "But the Helper, the Holy Spirit, whom the Father will send in My name, He will teach you all things, and bring to your remembrance all things that I said to you." Jesus also says, in Jhn 16:13, "Howbeit when he, the Spirit of truth, is come, he will guide you into all truth..."

I share these Scriptures to support my assertion that the Holy Spirit was the one who prompted me to question the pastor's interpretation of the verses from Hebrews. I believe He reminded me (brought to my "remembrance") of other Scriptures that had a different explanation of the "promises" that these great men and women of faith in Hebrews chapter 11 didn't receive.

Almost instantly, the Holy Spirit told me that the promise these Old Testament faith greats didn't receive was the promise of the Messiah. After this prompting by the Holy Spirit, I began to study to show myself approved and "not be ashamed" that I hadn't "rightfully divided" the Word, the passages in question. My opinion means nothing. I have no response to what that pastor or anyone else teaches other than the Word of God.

At the Holy Spirit's prompting, I went back like the Bereans and studied the Scriptures to see if what that pastor said was true. I was also motivated because I had never heard this particular argument against healing. The pastor had tied healing to prosperity teachers and false teaching.

His strong stance made me more eager to find the Scriptures to disprove his words. Studying to prove him wrong would be an improper motivation all by itself, but I had to follow the leading of the Holy Spirit and find Scripture to support what I believed.

When I studied the Scriptures to find out what the promises in Heb 11: 13 and 39-40 were related to, I was surprised at what I found. I wasn't surprised because I found some connection to healing. Nothing I found in my study even indirectly implied that the passages in Hebrews related to God's healing promises. What surprised me was the promises related to so much more than the coming Messiah!

The promises the Old Testament saints such as Abel, Enoch, Noah, and Abraham (Heb 11:4-13, 20-39) "saw from afar off" but never received, pertained to the coming of the Messiah, restoration of Israel, resurrection and ascension of the Messiah, all enemies placed at the feet of the Messiah, the promise of eternal life, and the gift of the Holy Ghost.

I found Scripture after Scripture in just a few moments of searching online, confirming what these "unfulfilled promises" were. Why, then, did this pastor come up with his interpretation of these verses?

As I stated previously, I believe that his experience of having a loved one die was so powerful and overwhelming that it clouded his doctrine. Perhaps his experience blinded him to the point where he could not see the truth of Scripture in this area. Or he was hindered to the point where he could no longer search the Scripture to support a premise different from the one in his heart. The force of his personal experience was so powerful that it made him bend this Scripture to an interpretation that is totally unrelated to healing.

That's why God tells us to study. Scriptures can knowingly and unknowingly be twisted to support just about anything. But we don't have to study Scripture on our own. We have the Holy Spirit, the Helper, the One who leads us into all truth, the One who reminds us of the things that Jesus said. The Bible says of God the Holy Spirit that "He bears witness with our spirit." From Strong's definition, that means the Holy Spirit "testifies," "corroborates evidence." (Blue Letter Bible, n.d.)

A witness is someone who saw something. In Jhn 16:13, the Bible says of the Holy Spirit that "he will guide you into all truth: for he shall not speak of himself; but whatsoever he shall hear, that shall he speak." The Holy Spirit only speaks what He has seen and heard from the Father.

We can trust the leading of the Spirit because He leads us based on what He has heard from the Father. If you want a greater understanding of what it means to listen to the Holy Spirit and hear the voice of God, please see my books "Lifesaving the Importance of Hearing the Voice of God" and "Lifesaving Vol II Hardening Your Heart to the Voice of God."

Everything I said may sound pretty convincing. But we must learn to take the extra step to confirm everything we believe or base our doctrine upon in Scripture. This key spiritual principle is established in 2 Tim 3:16: "All scripture is given by inspiration of God, and is profitable for doctrine, for reproof, for correction, for instruction in righteousness."

I will share the Scriptures I found, and in some cases, I will add a note to show how it supports what I believe these unfulfilled promises were. Again, nothing in these Scriptures points even remotely to God's healing promises, God's will to heal, etc.

"Then the one whose name was Cleopas answered and said to Him, 'Are You the only stranger in Jerusalem, and have You not known the things which happened there in these days?' And He said to them, 'What things?' So they said to Him, 'The things concerning Jesus of Nazareth, who was a Prophet mighty in deed and word before God and all the people, and how the chief priests and our rulers delivered

Him to be condemned to death, and crucified
Him. <u>But we were hoping that it was He who was
going to redeem Israel</u>....

Behold, I send <u>the Promise of My Father</u> upon
you; but tarry in the city of Jerusalem until you
are endued with power from on high."

*The Promise of My Father here was the Holy
Ghost as we will see in Acts.
*The phrase "we were hoping that it was He that
was going to redeem Israel" indicates one of the
promises that God had made that still was yet to
come

Luk 24:18-21, 49

"And, being assembled together with them,
commanded them that they should not depart
from Jerusalem, <u>but wait for the promise of the
Father</u>, which, saith he, ye have heard of me. For
John truly baptized with water; but ye shall be
baptized with <u>the Holy Ghost</u> not many days
hence. When they therefore were come
together, they asked of him, saying, Lord, wilt
thou at this time <u>restore again the kingdom to
Israel</u>? And he said unto them, It is not for you to
know the times or the seasons, which the Father
hath put in his own power. But ye shall receive

power, after that <u>the Holy Ghost</u> is come upon you: and ye shall be witnesses unto me both in Jerusalem, and in all Judaea, and in Samaria, and unto the uttermost part of the earth."

Act 1:4-8

"But Peter, standing up with the eleven, raised his voice and said to them, 'Men of Judea and all who dwell in Jerusalem, let this be known to you, and heed my words. For these are not drunk, as you suppose, since it is only the third hour of the day. But <u>this is what was spoken by the prophet Joel</u>: '<u>And it shall come to pass in the last days, says God, That I will pour out of My Spirit on all flesh</u>; Your sons and your daughters shall prophesy, Your young men shall see visions, Your old men shall dream dreams. And on My menservants and on My maidservants I will pour out My Spirit in those days; And they shall prophesy. I will show wonders in heaven above And signs in the earth beneath: Blood and fire and vapor of smoke. The sun shall be turned into darkness, And the moon into blood, before the coming of the great and awesome day of the Lord. And it shall come to pass that whoever calls on the name of the Lord Shall be saved.'"

Act 2:14-21

*The prophet Joel saw afar off, if you will, the promised pouring out of the Holy Spirit but never received himself. Joel saw the "great and awesome day of the Lord" and other last-days manifestations mentioned in this passage that we have still yet to see.

"Men of Israel, hear these words: Jesus of Nazareth, a Man attested by God to you by miracles, wonders, and signs which God did through Him in your midst, as you yourselves also know—Him, being delivered by the determined purpose and foreknowledge of God, you have taken by lawless hands, have crucified, and put to death; whom God raised up, having loosed the pains of death, because it was not possible that He should be held by it. For David says concerning Him: 'I foresaw the LORD always before my face, For He is at my right hand, that I may not be shaken. Therefore my heart rejoiced, and my tongue was glad; Moreover my flesh also will rest in hope. For You will not leave my soul in Hades, Nor will You allow Your Holy One to see corruption. You have made known to me the ways of life; You will make me full of joy in Your presence.'"

Act 2:22-28

*Through the power of the Holy Spirit, David "foresaw" (saw afar off) the promised Savior, saw that he would be resurrected and not left in Hades, that the Savior would not see "corruption" and that one day he (David) would be full of joy in His presence. David did not live to see these promises because the time for their fulfillment had not yet come.

"Fellow children of Abraham and you God-fearing Gentiles, it is to us that this message of salvation has been sent. The people of Jerusalem and their rulers did not recognize Jesus, yet in condemning him they fulfilled the words of the prophets that are read every Sabbath. Though they found no proper ground for a death sentence, they asked Pilate to have him executed. When they had carried out all that was written about him, they took him down from the cross and laid him in a tomb. But God raised him from the dead, and for many days he was seen by those who had traveled with him from Galilee to Jerusalem. They are now his witnesses to our people. "We tell you the good news: <u>What God promised our ancestors</u> he has fulfilled for us, their children, by raising up

Jesus. As it is written in the second Psalm: 'You are my son; today I have become your father.' God raised him from the dead so that <u>he will never be subject to decay</u>. As God has said, 'I will give you the holy and sure blessings promised to David.' So it is also stated elsewhere: 'You will not let your holy one see decay.' 'Now when David had served God's purpose in his own generation, he fell asleep; he was buried with his ancestors and his body decayed. But the one whom God raised from the dead did not see decay."

Act 13:26-37

*In this passage, we see two promises that weren't fulfilled for the Old Testament saints: the coming of the Messiah, Jesus, and the promise that the Messiah would be raised from the dead and not see decay.

"Now, fellow Israelites, I know that you acted in ignorance, as did your leaders. But this is <u>how God fulfilled what he had foretold through all the prophets</u>, saying that his Messiah would suffer. Repent, then, and turn to God, so that your sins may be wiped out, that times of refreshing may come from the Lord, and that he may send the Messiah, who has been appointed for you—even Jesus. 21 Heaven must receive him <u>until the time comes</u> <u>for God to restore everything, as he promised long ago through his holy prophets</u>. For Moses said, 'The Lord your God will raise up for you a prophet like me from among your own people; you must listen to everything he tells you. Anyone who does not listen to him will be completely cut off from their people.'"

Act 3:17-23

"And behold, there was a man in Jerusalem whose name was Simeon, and this man was just and devout, waiting for the Consolation of Israel, and the Holy Spirit was upon him. And <u>it had been revealed to him by the Holy Spirit that he would not see death before he had seen the Lord's Christ</u>. So he came by the Spirit into the temple. And when the parents brought in the Child Jesus, to do for Him according to the custom of the law, he took Him up in his arms and blessed God and said: 'Lord, now You are letting Your servant depart in peace,
According to Your word; For my eyes have seen Your salvation which You have prepared before the face of all peoples, A light to bring revelation

to the Gentiles, And the glory of Your people
Israel.'"

*I shared this Scripture to show that in the
fullness of time, God sent forth His Son (Gal 4:4).
Jesus was promised to the Old Testament saints,
but the fulfillment of the promise was set for a
later time, as witnessed by Simeon.

"Does this blessedness then come upon the
circumcised only, or upon the uncircumcised
also? For we say that faith was accounted to
Abraham for righteousness. How then was it
accounted? While he was circumcised, or
uncircumcised? Not while circumcised, but while
uncircumcised. And he received the sign of
circumcision, a seal of the righteousness of the
faith which he had while still uncircumcised,
that he might be the father of all those who
believe, though they are uncircumcised, that
righteousness might be imputed to them
also, and the father of circumcision to those who
not only are of the circumcision, but who also
walk in the steps of the faith which our
father Abraham had while still uncircumcised.
For the promise that he would be the heir of the

world was not to Abraham or to his seed
through the law, but through the righteousness
of faith. For if those who are of the law are heirs,
faith is made void and the promise made of no
effect, because the law brings about wrath; for
where there is no law there is no transgression.
Therefore it is of faith that it might be according
to grace, <u>so that the promise might be sure to all
the seed, not only to those who are of the law,
but also to those who are of the faith of
Abraham, who is the father of us all</u>

Rom 4:9-16

*The promise that Abraham would be "heir of
the world" included the Gentiles who became
righteous through faith in Christ. Because Christ
had not yet come, Abraham did not receive the
fulfillment of this promise while he was on earth.

"that the blessing of Abraham might come upon
the Gentiles in Christ Jesus, that we might
receive the promise of the Spirit through faith."

Gal 3:14

"But the Scripture has confined all under sin,
that the promise by faith in Jesus Christ might be
given to those who believe."

Gal 3:22

"that the Gentiles should be fellow heirs, of the
same body, and partakers of His promise in
Christ through the gospel..."

Eph 3:6

"So do not throw away your confidence; it will
be richly rewarded. You need to persevere so
that when you have done the will of God, you
will receive what he has promised."

Heb 10:35-36 (NIV)

"Beloved, I now write to you this second epistle
(in both of which I stir up your pure minds by
way of reminder), that you may be mindful of
the words which were spoken before by the holy
prophets, and of the commandment of us, the
apostles of the Lord and Savior, knowing this
first: that scoffers will come in the last
days, walking according to their own lusts, and

saying, "Where is the promise of His coming? For
since the fathers fell asleep, all things continue
as they were from the beginning of creation...

But, beloved, do not forget this one thing, that
with the Lord one day is as a thousand years,
and a thousand years as one day. The Lord is not
slack concerning His promise, as some count
slackness, but is longsuffering toward us, not
willing that any should perish but that all should
come to repentance. But the day of the Lord will
come as a thief in the night, in which the
heavens will pass away with a great noise, and
the elements will melt with fervent heat; both
the earth and the works that are in it will
be burned up. Therefore, since all these things
will be dissolved, what manner of persons ought
you to be in holy conduct and godliness, looking
for and hastening the coming of the day of God,
because of which the heavens will be dissolved,
being on fire, and the elements will melt with
fervent heat? Nevertheless we, according to His
promise, look for new heavens and a new earth
in which righteousness dwells."

2 Pet 3:1-4, 8-10 (NKJV)

*The Old Testament saints were promised, and
many saw by the power of the Holy Spirit the
day of the Lord Jesus' return. We, too, have the

same promise and the promise of a "new heaven and a new earth." These promises have yet to be fulfilled.

"Therefore let that abide in you which you heard from the beginning. If what you heard from the beginning abides in you, you will also abide in the Son and the Father. <u>And this is the promise that He has promised us—eternal life</u>."

I Jhn 2 (NKJV)

We know that God made a promise to restore Israel. We see that in Act 1:6-7: "Therefore, when they had come together, they asked Him, saying, 'Lord, will You at this time restore the kingdom to Israel?' And He said to them, It is not for you to know times or seasons which the Father has put in His own authority.'" This was a promise that the Old Testament saints never saw in their lifetime.

I did a brief search for Scriptures where God promised the restoration of Israel, but there was too much to digest and try to incorporate in this chapter. I share the Scriptures below as a potential starting point for further study for those who would desire to do so.

"Know and understand this: From the time the word goes out to restore and rebuild Jerusalem until the Anointed One, the ruler, comes, there will be seven 'sevens,' and sixty-two 'sevens.' It will be rebuilt with streets and a trench, but in times of trouble.

Dan 9:25 (NIV)

"He will set up a banner for the nations, And will assemble the outcasts of Israel, And gather together the dispersed of Judah From the four corners of the earth."

Isa 11:12 (NKJV)

"For the LORD will have mercy on Jacob, and will still choose Israel, and settle them in their own land. The strangers will be joined with them, and they will cling to the house of Jacob."

Isa 14:1 (NKJV)

"But Israel shall be saved by the LORD With an everlasting salvation; You shall not be ashamed or disgraced Forever and ever."

Isa 45:17 (NKJV)

The Power to Choose Life

"See, I set before you today life and
prosperity, death and destruction. For I
command you today to love the Lord your God,
to walk in obedience to him, and to keep his
commands, decrees and laws; then you will
live and increase, and the Lord your God will
bless you in the land you are entering to possess.
But if your heart turns away and you are not
obedient, and if you are drawn away to bow
down to other gods and worship them, I declare
to you this day that you will certainly be
destroyed. You will not live long in the land you
are crossing the Jordan to enter and possess.
This day I call the heavens and the Earth as
witnesses against you that I have set before you
life and death, blessings and curses. Now choose
life, so that you and your children may live and
that you may love the Lord your God, listen to
his voice, and hold fast to him. For the Lord is
your life, and he will give you many years in the
land he swore to give to your fathers, Abraham,
Isaac and Jacob."

Deu 30:15-20 (NIV)

The questions of why God allows suffering and doesn't answer some prayers seem to pop up repeatedly in books. On the surface, they seem like excellent questions. But often, they are based on a faulty, even demonic, premise.

When I say demonic, I do so to indicate the source and intent. In the Garden of Eden, Satan suggested to Adam and Eve that God wasn't good, that He was withholding something good from them.

The devil has no new tricks. The devil still asserts today that God isn't inherently and infinitely good and that He withholds good things from us or allows evil things to happen to us.

The Bible says that if Adam and Eve ate from the forbidden tree's fruit, they would gain the knowledge of good and evil. But the devil tricked Adam and Eve into rebelling against God primarily by getting them to believe God was withholding something good.

In Genesis, the devil is identified as an orchestrator of evil, a choreographer of bad things in the lives of humans. But today, the devil, the father of lies, has somehow tricked humanity into associating evil things with a loving God. He has tricked humanity into quickly pointing the finger of blame at God for tragedies, untimely deaths, etc.

God has given us a Bible that tells us that the devil is a thief who comes to steal, kill, and destroy. Yet when something is stolen from us, killed, or destroyed, we are tricked into accusing God.

In Genesis, God describes the authorities on Earth. He identifies Himself as the ultimate authority in the universe and Adam as His delegated authority on Earth. The only thing Adam didn't have authority over were two trees in the garden. The tree of "the knowledge of good and evil" and the "tree of life." Nowhere in the early chapters of the book of Genesis does the Bible speak of Satan's authority.

We know from Scripture that Satan had great responsibility in Heaven when he was Lucifer. Jesus said He saw Satan "fall like lightning" when he was cast out of Heaven into the Earth (Luk 10:18). Yet Adam, not Satan, was given authority over the Earth.

Satan couldn't command Adam or Eve to do anything. But through deception and Adam and Eve's complicity, Satan was able to steal their authority, destroy their life in the garden, and ultimately kill them. Yes, kill them. Adam and Eve were supposed to live forever in the Garden of Eden. However, because they were deceived and sinned, they died instantly, spiritually, and later physically.

Why didn't God stop the serpent from tempting Eve? Or stop Adam from eating the fruit? Didn't God know the impact? Didn't God know what it would cost humanity and even His Son? The Bible says that we only know in part, but after we see Him face to face, we will know in full (1 Cor 13:9-12). We can't fully know why God allowed original sin or why He cast Satan and the third of the angels who fell into the Earth. But we do know that Adam was meant to have authority over them.

Before Adam and Eve ate from the tree, they were in total authority over the things on Earth (natural and spiritual). Adam had authority over every wild beast we could imagine: lions, tigers, leopards, alligators, and serpents.

There is no indication in Scripture that Adam was afraid of these creatures or built himself protection from them. Similarly, Adam wasn't afraid of the myriad of fallen angels on Earth. He didn't know about evil. Adam and Eve's obedience kept them from the knowledge of evil and under the perfect protection of God.

Only after Adam and Eve's sin do we begin to see lies, hiding, blaming, and murder. They opened a door in the Earth that Scripture says could not be closed until the arrival of the second Adam. Jesus the second

Adam, who walked the Earth but never sinned, was God's perfect backup plan. Backup plan?

God loved us so much that He wanted us to have free choice. The same free choice that all the angels, including Lucifer, had and abused. Jesus had the same free choice in Heaven when He left for Earth, humbled Himself, became born of a woman, and walked in flesh (Phi 2:6-8). The same choice Jesus had in the second garden, if you will, the Garden of Gethsemane, when He said, "nevertheless not my will but thine" (Luk 22:42). The same choice Jesus had when he decided not to call down "twelve legions of angels" to prevent His death on the cross (Mat 26:52-54).

I don't know why humanity having the power to choose is so important to God. Could it be that the best expression of love to our Father is a love given by choice? God knows that a powerful love made possible by choice also makes room for the choice of rejection.

The power of choice comes with the potential outcomes of theft, rape, murder, the creation of weapons, and every evil act of man. Man's power of choice made possible an evil so pervasive that it spread to every family on Earth except Noah's. Could God have wiped all humanity off the Earth and created beings incapable of choice? I don't know.

Perhaps the power of choice is an inseparable component of eternal spirits or souls and is what makes us different from dolphins, apes, etc. Whatever the reason, giving humanity the power to choose life with or without God was so important to God that He was willing to risk Jesus' death on the cross to make it possible.

So what does the power of choice have to do with suffering, sickness, and healing?

- We can choose not to go to the doctor or ignore his advice
- We can choose to misuse our bodies by overeating, smoking, drinking to excess, using drugs
- We can choose to drive under the influence
- We can choose to end our own lives or the lives of others
- We can choose as Lot's wife did during the destruction of Sodom and Gomorrah to long for the desires and lifestyle of the world and receive the resultant consequences (Gen 19:25-26) (Pro 1:22-32) (Pro 3:1-2, 7-8)
- We can choose to quit fighting a debilitating disease and go on to our Heavenly reward
- We can choose not to believe in the power of the Scriptures to produce healing in our bodies

- We can choose not to believe in eternal life or what
  the Bible says about how to obtain it (Jhn 3:15-19)
- We can choose to remain ignorant of the Scriptures
  and suffer consequences (Hosea 4:6 "My people are
  destroyed for lack of knowledge")
- We can choose to blindly follow or receive a
  preacher's words on the subject of healing instead
  of following the Biblical exhortations to: 1) "Study to
  shew thyself approved unto God, a workman that
  needeth not to be ashamed, rightly dividing the
  word of truth" (2 Tim 2:15), 2) receive the Word
  with gladness (Mar 4:16) but to search the
  Scriptures daily to see if what is being preached is
  true (Act 17:11)
- We can choose to rely on, put trust and confidence
  in the traditions of men and "make the word of God
  of no effect" of no delivering and healing power
  (Mar 7:13)
- We can choose to doubt the Word of God on healing
  and be like a wave tossed on the sea and expect to
  receive none of the promises connected to it (Jam
  1:6-7)
- We can choose to come to God, please Him with our
  faith, and "believe that He is and that He is a
  rewarder of those that diligently seek Him" (Heb
  11:6)

- We can take His Word and "mix it with faith" (Heb 4:2) and "through faith and patience receive His promises" (Heb 6:12)
- Many times Jesus said, "thy faith hath made thee whole" (Mat 9:22, Mat 15:28, Mar 5:34, Mar 10:52, Luk 7:50, Luk 8:48, Luk 17:19, Luk 18:42), or He indicated that someone's healing was in part connected to their belief, faith, or ability to believe "do you believe I am able to do this" etc. (Mat 9:28, Mar 9:23-24, Mar 11:23-24, Luk 8:50); choosing to believe is a vital component of receiving healing

Hopefully, you took the time to look up and meditate on the many Scriptures I have shared. I pray that you can see the potential impact of our choices on our health and the amount of suffering we might experience.

Heb 9:27 says, "And as it is appointed unto men once to die, but after this the judgment." Have you ever heard someone say, "It was his or her time to go?" The idea that we have an "appointed" or set time to die is a very important theological discussion. Hos 4:6 says that even God's people can perish for "lack of knowledge." Before I dive into this discussion, I wanted to share the Scriptures I found around the topic:

"To everything there is a season, a time for every purpose under heaven: a time to be born, and a time to die."

Ecc 3:1 -2

"Is there not an appointed time to man upon earth? are not his days also like the days of an hireling?"

Job 7:1

"Seeing his days are determined, the number of his months are with thee, thou hast appointed his bounds that he cannot pass."

Job 14:5

"For I know that thou wilt bring me to death, and to the house appointed for all living."

Job 30:23

"For I think that God hath set forth us the apostles last, as it were appointed to

death: for we are made a spectacle unto the
world, and to angels, and to men.”

1 Co 4:9

“Do not be overly wicked, Nor be foolish: Why
should you die before your time?”

Ecc 7:17 (NKJV)

For you created my inmost being; you knit me
together in my mother’s womb. I praise
you because I am fearfully and wonderfully
made; your works are wonderful, I know that full
well. My frame was not hidden from you when I
was made in the secret place, when I was woven
together in the depths of the earth. Your eyes
saw my unformed body; all the days
ordained for me were written in your book
before one of them came to be.

Psa 139:13-16 (NIV)

“In those days Hezekiah was sick and near death.
And Isaiah the prophet, the son of Amoz, went
to him and said to him, ‘Thus says the Lord: ‘Set
your house in order, for you shall die and not

live." Then Hezekiah turned his face toward the wall, and prayed to the Lord, and said, 'Remember now, O Lord, I pray, how I have walked before You in truth and with a loyal heart, and have done what is good in Your sight.' And Hezekiah wept bitterly. And the word of the Lord came to Isaiah, saying, "Go and tell Hezekiah, 'Thus says the Lord, the God of David your father: 'I have heard your prayer, I have seen your tears; surely I will add to your days fifteen years. I will deliver you and this city from the hand of the king of Assyria, and I will defend this city."

Isa 38:1-6

"And it happened, before Isaiah had gone out into the middle court, that the word of the Lord came to him, saying, 'Return and tell Hezekiah the leader of My people, 'Thus says the Lord, the God of David your father: 'I have heard your prayer, I have seen your tears; surely I will heal you..."

2 Ki 20:4-6

"The days of our years are threescore years and ten; and if by reason of strength they be fourscore years, yet is their strength labour and sorrow; for it is soon cut off, and we fly away."

Psa 90:10

"And the Lord said, "My Spirit shall not always strive with man, for he also is flesh; yet his days shall be a hundred and twenty years."

Gen 6:3

There is so much to unpack in these Scriptures related to whether or not there is an appointed or set time to die. I shared so many Scriptures because I believe Scriptural questions should be answered with Scripture. The Bible says in 2 Tim 3:16 that we establish our doctrine on Scripture, but many Bible commentaries, especially online where anyone can post one, often veer off into opinions.

I want to start with the last two Scriptures I shared from Psa 90:10 and Gen 6:3. These Scriptures suggest a range that our appointed time should be within. That range would be between "three score and 10" or 70 years and 120 years. I can already hear voices yelling everyone doesn't live 70 years!

If you start by throwing out the Scriptures that say we should live between 70 and 120 years, how can you turn to the other Scriptures to say we have an appointed time? All Scripture, properly interpreted, is valid, or it isn't.

We can't throw out Scripture because of our personal experience. In fact, we must always do the opposite. We must always rigorously question any personal experience that doesn't align with Scripture. 2 Tim 3:16 says that all the Scriptures are breathed by God, divinely inspired. We should never try to bring the Word of God down to the level of our personal experience. Whenever there is a disconnect between the two, we must dig deeper into the Word for more answers.

Who is more likely to be full of contradictions, God in Heaven, for whom it is impossible to lie, or us? The Bible says in 1 Cor 13:9-12 that while we are here on earth, "we know in part" and that our limited knowledge is like trying to see through a dark glass. The verses imply that we won't know or understand some things until we see God "face to face."

Our bodies are a gift, and neglecting our bodies is bad stewardship. There are consequences associated with poor stewardship of our bodies that cannot be blamed on God and lumped under the banner "it was his or her time to go." However, I believe God, in His mercy, can heal bodies that have been made sick through poor stewardship. In reading the healing accounts of Jesus, I don't see where He said I cant or won't heal you because you brought this on yourself.

I have already shared Scriptures that say we can live between 70 and 120 years. I have set my faith on becoming a centurion, a "triple-digit man." I believe living to 100 or more is possible because the Bible says it is. On the flip side, I also believe that I should live to be at least 70 or "threescore and ten."

If you believe that God sends sickness to "call people home" or because "He needed them more in Heaven" or some other tradition of man, you may allow the devil to steal years of your time here on Earth. The Bible says Jesus "went about doing good and healing all who were oppressed by the devil, for God was with Him" (Act 10:38). Jesus lengthened the lives of some of the people He healed. He even raised sick people from the dead (Lazarus Jhn 11:38-44, Jairus' daughter Mar 5:21-43).

I see this same principle in Hezekiah's life. He was sick, and God sent the great prophet Isaiah to tell Hezekiah that he was about to die and to get his affairs in order. Under the "when it's your time" type of thinking, there would be nothing Hezekiah could do. This interpretation fixes our death entirely upon God and, worse, mixes sickness and disease into God's calculation of when we should go.

> "For to me, to live is Christ and to die is gain. If I am to go on living in the body, this will mean fruitful labor for me. Yet what shall I choose? I do not know! I am torn between the two: I desire to depart and be with Christ, which is better by far; but it is more necessary for you that I remain in the body. Convinced of this, I know that I will remain, and I will continue with all of you for your progress and joy in the faith, so that through my being with you again your boasting in Christ Jesus will abound on account of me."

Phi 1:21-26

Satan shortened Adam and Eve's lives, spiritually and physically, because of their disobedience. Let's live the longest lives possible by being good stewards of our bodies, heeding doctors' warnings, by watching our words, and being obedient to the Holy Spirit.

The Power of Words

"Death and life are in the power of the tongue:
and they that love it shall eat the fruit thereof."

Pro 18:21

"A man shall eat good by the fruit of his
mouth..."

Pro 13:2 (NKJV)

"For as he thinks in his heart, so is he..."

Pro 23:7

"And they overcame him by the blood of the
Lamb, and by the word of their testimony; and
they loved not their lives unto the death."

Rev 12:11

"He that keepeth his mouth keepeth his
life: but he that openeth wide his lips shall have
destruction."

I have a relative who asks, "Do you have a cold? Are you sick?" every time I cough, sneeze, or sniffle. While it is true that coughing, sneezing, or sniffling are signs of a cold or flu, sometimes they are not. I usually wake up with sniffles if I sleep directly under a fan or in the direct line of sight of the air conditioner.

Like many of us, this relative has been conditioned to label symptoms. I am tempted to do the same. I'm 58. My mom has bad arthritis. So did her mom. When I have pain in the bones of my hand, there is a temptation to say, "Maybe I have arthritis" vs. "I'm having some pain in my hand." Some of this comes from medical science. Medical science takes symptoms and tries to match them to known disease categories.

Years ago, decades ago, a doctor tried to tell me that my low white blood cell count might be leukemia or some other horrible disease. I nicknamed him "Dr. Gloom and Doom" because he chose to focus on the worst possible outcomes for my symptoms. I chose not to believe the worst. I'm not saying that the doctor couldn't have been right. If he had, I would have directed my faith toward the correctly diagnosed disease.

About 15-20 years ago, I had blood in my urine, and the doctor said, "You probably have cancer. Blood in the urine is usually a sign of cancer, or you may have..." Like "Dr. Gloom and Doom," he led off with the worst possible outcomes in a very matter-of-fact way. He might have gotten an "A" in his science classes, but he definitely would get an "F" in beside manner.

The doctor's job is to diagnose and match symptoms to known disease categories. My job is to listen to his words and prayerfully consider them. Before you conclude that I don't believe in doctors or medical science, please read the chapter in Healing Promises Vol I entitled "Go to the Doctor/Take Your Medicine."

All I'm saying is that you should be careful about what you say and what you agree with. If the doctor is not 100% sure, why should I agree with his worst possible outcome? Even if I didn't have faith in God, I would get a second or perhaps a third opinion.

At the start of the chapter, I show the importance the Bible places on our words. We were created in the image of God as speaking spirits with authority in our words. God, "the Father of Spirits" (Heb 12:9), spoke the universe into being. God gave Adam the power to speak and name.

In the Garden of Eden, God told Adam to use his words and name the animals; whatever Adam named them, that's what they were. Adam also named Eve:

"Out of the ground the Lord God formed every beast of the field and every bird of the air, and brought them to Adam to see what he would call them. And whatever Adam called each living creature, that was its name."

Gen 2:19 (NKJV)

"Adam named his wife Eve, because she would become the mother of all the living."

Gen 3:20 (NIV)

Our words have tremendous power. Pro 12:18 says, "The words of the reckless pierce like swords, but the tongue of the wise brings healing." Eph 4:29 says, "Do not let any unwholesome talk come out of your mouths, but only what is helpful for building others up according to their needs, that it may benefit those who listen." Even secular research confirms the power of negative words.

Researchers have proven that words spoken to children, such as "You'll never amount to anything," "You're no better than your father," "You're so stupid," etc., can cripple a child mentally and emotionally. In secular circles, we would call that type of treatment verbal abuse. The term "verbal abuse" recognizes that words can cause harm. Verbally abused children can grow up with insecurities and other psychological impairments simply because they were forced to sit under the wrong words.

We can understand that a child might not have the mental and emotional capability to resist the negative words that are spoken into them. I'm using the word "into" because Pro 12:18 says that words can pierce our souls.

The image that comes to mind is a child forced to sit, with an open mouth, under a fountain of tainted water as it is poured into their soul. In the military, they have a form of torture called waterboarding. The tortured person is forced to endure having harmful amounts of water poured down their throat.

Verbally abused children are forced to consciously or subconsciously agree with their parents' words. They internalize these negative words and the accompanying psychological and emotional harm.

That's no different to me than my choosing to agree with the words spoken over me by the relative who wanted me to agree with her that I was sick because I had sniffles. That was her assessment or diagnosis of my symptoms. As an adult, I understand I don't have to agree with her words, so they have no power over me. Also, as someone with a Scriptural revelation about the power of words, I understand the consequences of agreeing with her words.

In the spiritual realm, if I agree with her words, I give them supernatural power over me and open a door for sickness and disease to operate legally in my body. More on that in a moment.

What about the words you say to yourself? Comments like, "I always get sick this time of year," and "My mother and father had diabetes, so I guess I will too." Most people have heard the phrase negative self-talk. Even people who are not spiritual would likely agree that it is harmful to say things like "I'm just a screwup," "I'll never be able to lose weight," "I wasn't born into the right social class or race, so I don't have much chance for success in life." There is a multi-billion-dollar industry that markets positive self-talk and self-image books, videos, seminars, etc., to address harmful self-talk.

Why don't we see that saying negative words about our health is harmful when we recognize the inherent power of saying other bad things about ourselves? Hos 4:6 says, "My people are destroyed for lack of knowledge."

We don't exercise special care with our words when we don't have the revelation that the words we say can impact our physical health just like they impact our mental and emotional health. We loosely say things like, "I'm really sick. It's probably pneumonia," or "I probably won't live to be 80; none of the men in my family made it past 75." Often, there is no one to disagree with us when we speak negative words about ourselves.

Pro 23:7 indicates that there is even some degree of power in our internal dialogue, what we think in our hearts. We can become what we think in our hearts. If we allow negative internal dialogue (e.g., "I will get arthritis like my mom did." or "I will die before 80 like the other men in my family) to build, it will overflow out of our mouths. Mat 12:34 (NKJV) says, "... For out of the abundance of the heart the mouth speaks.

Whether we come into agreement with negative words spoken over us or speak negative words over ourselves, a door is opened. Eph 4:25-27 (NKJV) says that we can do certain things that "give place to the devil" (give the devil a foothold-NIV).

"Therefore, putting away lying, 'Let each one of you speak truth with his neighbor,' for we are members of one another. 'Be angry, and do not sin': do not let the sun go down on your wrath, nor give place to the devil."

The Bible says our words can set things in motion in the spirit realm. Dan 10:12 (NKJV) says, "Then he said to me, "Do not fear, Daniel, for from the first day that you set your heart to understand, and to humble yourself before your God, your words were heard; and I have come because of your words." A supernatural being, an angel, was sent in response to Daniel's words. Here are some other examples of supernatural results from a man's words:

"Therefore confess your sins to each other and pray for each other so that you may be healed. The prayer of a righteous person is powerful and effective. Elijah was a human being, even as we are. He prayed earnestly that it would not rain, and it did not rain on the land for three and a half years. Again he prayed, and the heavens gave rain, and the earth produced its crops."

Jam 5:16-18 (NIVUK)

"And Elijah the Tishbite, of the inhabitants of Gilead, said to Ahab, "As the Lord God of Israel lives, before whom I stand, there shall not be dew nor rain these years, except at my word."

1 Ki 17:1 (NKJV)

"On the day the Lord gave the Amorites over to Israel, Joshua said to the Lord in the presence of Israel: "Sun, stand still over Gibeon, and you, moon, over the Valley of Aijalon."So the sun stood still, and the moon stopped, till the nation avenged itself on its enemies, as it is written in the Book of Jashar. The sun stopped in the middle of the sky and delayed going down about a full day. There has never been a day like it before or since, a day when the Lord listened to a human being. Surely the Lord was fighting for Israel!"

Jos 10:12-14

Our words spoken in faith can move God and His angels (Psa 103:20-21). The devil can also use them in negative ways. Just like the words you say in police custody or on the witness stand can be used against you

in courts on earth, the words you speak can be used
against you in the spiritual realm, in the courts of
Heaven:

"Then I heard a loud voice saying in heaven,
'Now salvation, and strength, and the kingdom
of our God, and the power of His Christ have
come, for the accuser of our brethren, who
accused them before our God day and night, has
been cast down.'"

Rev 12:10

"Be sober, be vigilant, because your adversary
the devil walketh about as a roaring lion, seeking
whom he may devour."

1 Pet 5:8

"Hereafter I will not talk much with you: for the
prince of this world cometh, and hath nothing in
me."

Jhn 14:30

Imagine the devil walking around in the spiritual realm, seeking to catch words that he can use against us and accuse us before God. The Bible says that day and night, he accuses us before God.

Jesus said in Jhn 14:30 that Satan had nothing in Him. I know this dealt primarily with sin, but I believe it also included His words. Jesus gave no place to the devil through His actions or His words.

I Prayed and They Died

I know what it's like to stand in prayer for someone who died. I know what it's like to pray for someone and see healings, even those that don't make sense to the doctors. I can imagine the grief that someone might experience who prayed for a loved one who didn't get better and died. I can imagine how that might affect their ability to believe in Scriptures related to healing.

On the other hand, what hope do we have if everything in the Bible isn't true? I'm writing this book to stir your hope and faith. I hope to rekindle the flame of your hope if it has been blown out due to the death of a loved one. The death of a loved one is likely one of the greatest pains a person can experience. It can be so powerful that it can change everything you believe about God and maybe even weaken your will to continue living.

The only remedy I know is to press deeper into the Word of God until it begins to become larger than the loss you have experienced. We can never let what we have experienced become a greater truth than the written Word of God. I have learned from years of studying sermons and books from some of the greatest Bible teachers that faith is a tool.

Yes, faith is a tool that can be used as a weapon. If you've ever seen kids play the video game "Call of Duty," you have seen them level up or enhance their weapons. Faith is a tool, a weapon that can be enhanced and grow more powerful. Like in the video game, faith is a weapon that must be recharged. Faith is recharged by hearing God's Word and "studying to show yourself approved."

Faith is a weapon that must be tested in battle. When King Saul gave David his armor, David said no, "I haven't proven these." David went to fight Goliath with weapons he had proven in killing a lion and a bear. I have learned from Gloria Copeland that, unfortunately, some people run out to face cancer with faith and Scriptures they haven't proven against the flu.

When confronted by the devil in the wilderness, Jesus didn't have to search for Scriptures. He could stand in faith and respond, "It is written..." skillfully with Scriptures appropriate to every attack the devil launched.

When I was learning to play "Call of Duty," I remember my player being stabbed to death while holding an automatic weapon. As a player, I had a powerful weapon but didn't know how to use it properly.

Some people may have read that last paragraph and become offended, thinking I was saying that if their loved one died, it's because they didn't have the knowledge of the Scriptures or didn't have enough faith. I don't know that to be true of your loved one. But I do know that it is possible. Jesus rebuked the apostles for their lack of faith when they could not heal a boy that an evil spirit kept throwing into the fire.

I have seen people decide to stop fighting a terrible disease and go on to their eternal reward. Sometimes, they say they are "ready to go," and sometimes, they don't say it, but they have decided in their heart. I have seen people trust the Word to a point but ultimately believe the doctor's words more and don't make it. These were people that I cared about.

There are so many reasons that a person might not receive their healing. I dive into many of those in Healing Promises Vol I and, to some degree, in this book. I don't pretend to know all the reasons; only God does. I believe in the Word of God and its possibilities more than the deaths of the people I knew.

I am grateful to the Almighty God that I have also seen healings. Jesus said, "Blessed are they that have not seen yet believe (Jhn 20:29)." I have seen people follow the Scriptures in faith and be healed or live a lot longer than the doctors expected.

I wrote the first book for my 2nd mom, Earnestine Anderson. I wrote it because of the Holy Spirit's powerful and urgent prompting. Sometime after I had finished the book, I found out she had congestive heart failure.

I can testify to the healing power of God in her life. I know that the excess water in her lungs and heart went away and that she outlived the predictions of someone with that disease. However, I also know that she went to a church that believed God was behind the deaths of His saints and "plucks flowers from His garden" or gives "early graduations."

I can see why the Holy Spirit had me write an entire book for her and give her infusions of the Word. The Bible says the traditions of men make the Word of God of no effect. I could rephrase that and say if we believe things said from the pulpit that contradict the Word of God, we can render the most powerful weapon in the universe totally ineffective.

People can indeed believe the Bible, go to church every Wednesday night and Sunday morning and hear from the pulpit that the words in the Bible aren't true for some reason. Then, when it is time to use the weapon of the Word in a life-or-death battle, the weapon misfires.

It gets jammed by doubt that came not from the devil but from the pulpit. It's one of the reasons I have been so determined to include as many Scripture references as I can in this book and the previous one so that Christians can be armed with the truth.

In February 2022, I got a call from the hospice nurse. He said that my Dad was in imminent danger of having a stroke, heart failure, etc., because he had stopped taking his insulin for diabetes and his blood pressure medication.

My sisters, stepmom, a nurse, and I had an intervention with my Dad and asked him if he was trying to go on to his heavenly reward. He wasn't eating. He wasn't taking the medications I mentioned. He was barely drinking water. He had lost about 100 pounds. He was frail and showed the signs of "transition" identified in the hospice pamphlet.

My Dad had previously experienced full cardiac arrest and had to be resuscitated a few years earlier. He had also survived multiple heart attacks and a quadruple bypass in 2012. He survived COVID (no symptoms! In 2021). We did not think he would make it to his 80th birthday on Feb 8th, 2022.

I was prepared for my Dad to go. My sister and stepmom had made some preliminary arrangements.

Though I was prepared for him to go, I asked him to stay.

I was reminded of my workout partner, who told me a story about his mom. She was battling terminal cancer and had stopped eating and taking meds. He lied to her and told her his girlfriend was pregnant. She started taking her meds as well as eating and fighting again. My workout partner wasn't a Christian, and his mom eventually died, but there was a will to live, a desire to keep fighting that extended her life that I don't know how to quantify.

I believe my Dad rekindled his will to live and keep fighting. I also know that my Dad knows the Word. I gave him a healing book by Gloria Copeland many years ago. I took him to faith seminars in Los Angeles under Dr. Fredrick K. C. Price and in Maryland under Dr. Mike Freeman. I gave him a copy of the first book I wrote in this series. I have read Scriptures to him. One of my sisters is a minister and feeds him Scriptures and has prayed for him.

I asked my Dad to stick around until my first grandchild was born in April 2023. It is now September of 2023. He is still in hospice. He is bedridden and battling dementia and depression in a nursing home, but he is still here.

My Dad told me years ago, he overheard a doctor talking to a nurse about a picture of his heart, thinking it was someone deceased. The doctor was so embarrassed when my Dad spoke up and said those were his records. The point is my Dad is still fighting, and I believe the combination of his faith and his fight is why he is still here despite all the medical predictions.

I will continue to believe the Word of God first over my personal experiences, but I do believe some of my personal experiences result from what I believe. I have experienced many healings. I have been supernaturally healed of Irritable Bowel Syndrome (IBS) and Gastroesophageal Reflux Disease (GERD). I have been healed of several sports injuries: hernia, broken back, knee injuries, foot injuries, and, most recently, a torn rotator cuff. Surgery was prescribed for nearly all of these injuries, but I decided to test my faith.

Was I willing to get the surgery if praying and standing in faith "didn't work?" Of course. But glory to God, I was able to prove my faith in these small situations. I pray that I don't have to use it in a life-threatening situation. I have seen fevers broken when I laid my hands on my children. I have seen an outbreak of a virus dry up when my wife and I prayed.

Finally, I have heard the testimonies of people who have read the first book. One woman I knew from a show I did in Phoenix. Her husband had died, and she had two terminal diseases. She had cancer and some viral condition local to that area that the doctors felt would kill her first.

She was discouraged because her husband had died in the hospital. She told me he died believing some of the same Scriptures I had shared with her. I took a chance and asked her to tell me more about the circumstances surrounding her husband's death.

Often, I have found that there is more to the story than "faith just doesn't work." This was true in the case of her husband. He had gone into the hospital for routine surgery, something minor. However, he told her he didn't think he'd make it out of there. She didn't understand why he would say that for a minor procedure.

Her husband didn't make it out of the hospital. He caught an infection and died. I was able to carefully talk to her about the Scripture, "Death and life are in the power of the tongue," and the power of her husband's words.

It helped restore her faith, and I believe it helped her beat both the viral disease and the cancer. She believes that as well. Though I haven't talked to her, I also believe it helped her defeat cancer again when it returned a few years ago.

Her husband passed away, I believe, because of a door he opened with his words. I talk about that in Volume I. But hope is for the living. I believe her husband would have wanted her to keep hoping and trusting in the Word and power of God versus succumbing to a horrible, destructive death by cancer.

She told me that reading my book gave her hope. She had given up. That hope caused her to fight and led to our meeting, and she mixed the clarity she received with her faith and is still alive.

I wrote the first book for my mom, but this woman's testimony proved that God had an even greater purpose for that book. My natural mom has read it. Many others have read it or listened to it. I have seen other testimonies online in reviews.

I hope many will also read this book and be further encouraged in their faith to fight off disease and be built up against future attacks/diseases.

Happy Ending

Don't we get sad when the hero dies or squirm if the villain lives? If the villain lives, don't we assume there will be a sequel in which the villain will die? We all like stories with "happy" endings. The film industry has a familiar phrase called the "Hollywood ending." It refers to the hero riding off in the sunset, the girl getting rescued and marrying the prince, and the bad guy getting defeated. The truth is that the happy ending didn't originate in Hollywood.

"Now as Jesus passed by, He saw a man who was blind from birth. And His disciples asked Him, saying, "Rabbi, who sinned, this man or his parents, that he was born blind?" Jesus answered, 'Neither this man nor his parents sinned, but that the works of God should be revealed in him. I must work the works of Him who sent Me while it is day; the night is coming when no one can work. As long as I am in the world, I am the light of the world.' When He had said these things, He spat on the ground and made clay with the saliva; and He anointed the eyes of the blind man with the clay. And He said to him, 'Go, wash in the pool of Siloam' (which is translated, Sent). So he went and washed, and came back seeing."

Jhn 9:1-7

In an earlier chapter, we looked at the man in John chapter 9 who was born blind. The start of this man's story was bleak. He was born blind. The other characters in this story, the disciples, assumed the cause of the man's blindness was sin, either his or his parents.

The implication was that blindness was the end of the story—the man got the sin penalty that he deserved. Jesus wasn't satisfied with that ending of the man's story. The other implication was that the blindness was from God, God's punishment for sin. Jesus wasn't on board with that assessment, either.

Jesus tells the disciples that sin did not cause the man's blindness. Jesus said the blindness was there "that works of God should be revealed in him." 1 Jhn 3:8 says, "… For this purpose the Son of God was manifested, that he might destroy the works of the devil." Putting the two together, we see that this man's blindness served to reveal Jesus' purpose and work of destroying the works of the devil. God didn't send or cause the blindness but knew that this man would encounter Jesus and receive the "happy ending" to his story.

The healing of the blind man brought glory to the Father. The glorious part of the story is that God made provision for the man to be healed through a man with the knowledge of His healing power and equipped by the Spirit of God.

What if that was God's purpose for everyone born blind or lame? What if God's plan for them was to encounter men and women of faith and power who could lay hands on them, pray, and manifest their healing? We saw God manifest healing in the Old Testament and later, through Jesus, the Apostles, Paul, and Stephen.

The devil has twisted this parable not only to get us comfortable seeing people lame or otherwise disabled from birth but to label it as God's will! If we associate all birth defects, deformities, and sickness with God's will, there will be no motivation to pray for healing or miracles.

What if there was a drug or surgery that could reverse blindness or deafness, or a crippled hand? We have already seen surgeries that can remedy a cleft palate or other deformities. We applaud these man-made reversals of birth defects. Through knowledge gained in the study of medicine, we can prevent certain birth defects by telling pregnant women to avoid alcohol or drugs.

Gloria Copeland used to say if we really believed that a sickness (I'll add deformity) was the will of God and brought glory to God, why would we go to the doctor to get that "glory" off? The truth is that we really don't believe that. Deep down inside, we know that sickness is bad. We just don't know how to get rid of it, and we are likely more familiar with the remedies offered by modern medicine than the Bible.

A close friend of mine had a son, Caleb, who was born without an anus, and his arteries were routed to the wrong chambers of his heart. Through the "miracle" of modern medicine, a child survived that should have died in the first month of his life. Was it God's will that children like this die? Or was it in God's plan all along that medical discoveries would be made to eliminate these dreadful deformities?

I know in Caleb's case, it was not God's will that he should die in that first year of his life. In the first year of his life, God led me to send the parents birthday cards for his 2nd and 3rd birthdays. This was a prophetic act. I had never been led to do something like that before. Again, there was no expectation that Caleb would live to his first birthday.

He later was given HIV-infected blood in a transfusion (before current blood screening protocols became standard procedure). This infection further dimmed hopes that Caleb would live.

Caleb died of heart failure before his fourth birthday. I don't know why he later died after overcoming all the birth defects and the HIV-infected blood transfusion. I know that the God of the Universe knew He would live well beyond everything the doctors said.

The parents are dear friends who have been instrumental in my Christian walk. I think because of that we didn't talk about the birthday cards when I sent them. They didn't understand them at the time or their prophetic significance. We didn't discuss the birthday cards until years after Caleb's death. I am not propping myself up as a great prophet or man of God. All I knew was an incredible urgency to send these birthday cards.

I am trying to illustrate that the doctors' words aren't always the final words. God is still a God who performs miracles beyond any doctor's capability to explain. I believe God has helped men discover surgical procedures, vaccines, treatments, etc. He is the God of both the discovered and the undiscovered.

In this chapter, I hope to encourage you to believe for the "happy ending," whether it comes by God through the doctors' care or supernaturally through prayer and laying on of hands or some combination of the above.

I suffered a broken back at age 18 wrestling heavyweight, and after a word of knowledge (1 Cor 12:8) and a prayer on TV from Pat Robertson, I could do things from that day to age 58 that I previously couldn't do (no surgery required).

I want to see greater healings and miracles. The Bible says we can earnestly desire or covet these gifts. Perhaps we don't see more healings and miracles because more people aren't pursuing these gifts.

I want to manifest the works of Jesus (destroying the works of the devil) and the will of God (delivering people from the devil's work). I want to be the author of a happy ending for someone whose current circumstances say otherwise.

Self-Image and Healing

"Beloved, I pray that you may prosper in all things and be in health, just as your soul prospers."

3 Jhn 2 (NKJV)

"Every good gift and every perfect gift is from above, and cometh down from the Father of lights, with whom is no variableness, neither shadow of turning."

James 1:17

"Then the king said, 'Is there not still someone of the house of Saul, to whom I may show the kindness of God?' And Ziba said to the king, 'There is still a son of Jonathan who is lame in his feet.' So the king said to him, 'Where is he?' And Ziba said to the king, 'Indeed he is in the house of Machir the son of Ammiel, in Lo Debar.' Then King David sent and brought him out of the house of Machir the son of Ammiel, from Lo Debar. Now when Mephibosheth the son of Jonathan, the son of Saul, had come to David, he fell on his face and prostrated himself. Then David said, 'Mephibosheth?' And he answered, 'Here is your servant!' So David said to him, 'Do not fear, for I will surely show you kindness for Jonathan your father's sake, and will restore to you all the land of Saul your grandfather; and you shall eat bread at my table continually.' Then he bowed himself, and said, 'What is your servant, that you should look upon such a dead dog as I?' And the king called to Ziba, Saul's servant, and said to him, 'I have given to your master's son all that belonged to Saul and to all his house. You therefore, and your sons and your servants, shall work the land for him, and you shall bring in the harvest, that your master's son may have food to eat. But Mephibosheth your master's son shall eat bread at my table always.' Now Ziba had fifteen sons and twenty servants. Then Ziba said to the king, 'According to all that my lord the king has commanded his servant, so will your servant do.' 'As for Mephibosheth," said the king, "he shall eat at my table like one of the king's sons.'

2 Sam 9:3-11

"Let us therefore come boldly to the throne of grace, that we may obtain mercy and find grace to help in time of need."

Heb 4:16 (NKJV)

"'Come now, and let us reason together,' Says the Lord, 'though your sins are like scarlet, they shall be as white as snow.'"

Isa 1:18-20

One of the greatest obstacles to my healing has been my self-image. 3 Jhn 2 says, "Prosper and be in health even as your soul prospers." My former pastor, Dr. Mike Freeman, says you'll never prosper beyond the level of prosperity in your soul.

I didn't think I deserved anything good. That included career, family, success, health, or, at times, life. I am a survivor of physical, sexual, verbal, and spiritual abuse. These injuries crippled my concept of self-worth.

Only through the Scriptures and Christ-centered teaching have I become aware that I don't have to be worthy of receiving any manifestation of God's love (salvation, the Holy Spirit, gifts of the Spirit, healing, prosperity).

Growing in the revelation that my relationship with Jesus Christ makes me worthy is the key to receiving "every good and perfect gift" from the Father. Is there anything in your concept of worthiness that might be hindering your ability to receive God's healing, grace, and mercy?

You can't do anything to deserve any of God's gifts. Knowing that makes receiving them all the more powerful and inspires greater gratitude and love for God! Just receive His great gifts, knowing that they are a reflection of His greatness and goodness, not yours.

"The Lord is compassionate and gracious, slow to anger, abounding in love. He will not always accuse, nor will he harbor his anger forever; he does not treat us as our sins deserve or repay us according to our iniquities. For as high as the heavens are above the earth, so great is his love for those who fear him; as far as the east is from the west, so far has he removed our transgressions from us."

Psa 103: 8-12

Conclusion

"Praise the Lord, my soul; all my inmost being, praise his holy name. Praise the Lord, my soul, and forget not all his benefits— who forgives all your sins and heals all your diseases."

Psa 103:1-3

One time, I had something wrong with my car and discovered a vehicle recall had been issued. There was already a solution out there for my problem. I just didn't know it. The fact that I didn't know about it did not negate the existence of the solution. Scripture says to search for wisdom like "hidden treasure" (Pro 2:4). Can we say that in the area of healing, we have searched the Scriptures like they can answer life and death situations?

I have seen people search for medical answers like that, and I understand it. But which one are we relying on more? The best time to study Scriptures on healing is when you're healthy. I attended Gloria Copeland's Healing School twice at various Kenneth Copeland conventions.

She taught us to believe in God, walk in divine health, and pray to stay healthy. Most importantly, she urged us not to wait to study the Scriptures on healing and building up our faith for healing until after we have contracted a terminal illness. By then, it might be too late.

I have made it a point to follow the example of the Copelands, read books, and listen to sermons by the great healing evangelists. I have shared several of their names and ministry accounts in this book.

I have done my very best in this book to show that healing is God's will throughout the Bible. I have tried to show that though everyone we pray for may not get healed, we must continue to believe that God still heals today instead of bringing God and the Word down to the level of our experience. I have tried in two books to offer from my limited knowledge of the Bible some of the reasons people we pray for don't recover or receive healing.

I think it is fitting that I close the book with an admonition to the reader to be on guard for the devil, who will come to try to steal or choke off any revelation they have received in this book. Anticipate his actions. Reread the book or sections of the book as needed. Discuss the chapters with prayer partners.

"The sower sows the word. And these are the
ones along the path, where the word is sown:
when they hear, Satan immediately comes and
takes away the word that is sown in them. And
these are the ones sown on rocky ground: the
ones who, when they hear the word,
immediately receive it with joy. And they have
no root in themselves, but endure for a while;
then, when tribulation or persecution arises on
account of the word, immediately they fall away.
And others are the ones sown among thorns.
They are those who hear the word, but the cares
of the world and the deceitfulness of riches and
the desires for other things enter in and choke
the word, and it proves unfruitful. But those that
were sown on the good soil are the ones who
hear the word and accept it and bear
fruit, thirtyfold and sixtyfold and a hundredfold."

Mar 4:14-20

FINAL REFLECTIONS

Some time ago, I prayed for some people with
whom I had sent the audio version of Healing Promises
Vol I. As I was praying, I believe the Holy Spirit had me

pray against the devil's work to steal or choke the Word being sown in their hearts. I've never prayed that before.

I asked myself how some people could listen to Scriptures on healing or hear the Word preached on healing and still not get healed. I believe that question is answered in these Scriptures. We must guard against the devil's work to steal or choke off the Word sown in our hearts. That Word could be about healing or any other topic.

The devil is not worried about us hearing the Word per se. He knows the Bible says there are "forgetful hearers (Jam 1:25)." He knows that we must be doers of the Word, and the Word must be mixed with faith, and that patience has to be added to faith, and that faith without works is dead.

The devil's job is to steal the Word before we can mix it with faith. His job is to choke the Word before it can take root and produce a harvest of healing. Jam 1:6-8 (NKJV) says, "he who doubts is like a wave of the sea driven and tossed by the wind." Eph 4:14 says, "that we should no longer be children, tossed to and fro and carried about with every wind of doctrine."

Through the violent force of doubt and the tossing force of flawed doctrine and traditions of men, the devil keeps the word from taking root and producing a harvest in our lives. This is a form of spiritual warfare.

We must recognize that we are in a battle. There is a war going on. The devil is actively working against the growth of the Word that is sown in our hearts. We can't have the casual "word tossed by the wayside attitude" where we don't value the word. We must decide that we won't let what we hear get scattered.

I have an image of the devil's work to stop the Word of God from producing a harvest in our hearts. Like a bulldozer or earth mover, the devil pours piles of dirt, dirty unbelief, dirty doubt, dirty error, dirty confusion, dirty traditions, etc., on top of what is revealed to us in Scripture.

Revelation is a work of the Holy Spirit, and blinding is a work of the god of this world. Without the revelation of the Holy Spirit, you cannot overcome the blinding work of the god of this world. Do not allow yourself to be blinded to the revelation of healing in the Scriptures.

For those who read this book and are facing a crisis, I also recommend buying the audio version of Healing Promises Vol I on Audible to hear healing Scriptures throughout your day and even as you sleep. I close this book by sharing the testimony of a woman who did this:

"Linda 07-09-19

Comfort through the storms

This book has been a great help to me, I am
going through a physical challenge and at night
time when my mind should be resting I find I am
going through my greatest warfare. I began
listening to this book and the peace that it gives
is like medicine to my spirit, it helps me rest and
trust God, it reminds me of who I serve and who
I am. I highly recommend it, the writing is
excellent and the narrator is perfect for this
book. I listen to it 3 or 4 times a day, I sometimes
just play it as I am cooking like I would
background music because it builds up my
spirit."

Appendix A: Forty-two Miracles by Moses (Ex 7:10)

1. Moses' rod turned into a serpent (Ex 4:2-3).

2. The serpent was transformed into a rod (Ex 4:4).

3. Moses' hand was turned leprous (Ex 4:6).

4. Moses' hand was healed of leprosy (Ex 4:7).

5. The rod was turned into a serpent (Ex 4:30).

6. The serpent was turned into a rod (Ex 4:30).

7. Moses' hand was made leprous (Ex 4:30).

8. Moses' hand was healed of leprosy (Ex 4:30).

9. Moses' rod was turned into a serpent (Ex 7:9-10; magicians also did so, Ex 7:11-12).

10. Moses' rod swallowed the others (Ex 7:12).

11. The Nile River was changed into blood: first plague (Ex 7:14-25; the Egyptian magicians also did so, Ex 7:22).

12. He created frogs: second plague (Ex 8:1-7; the magicians also did so, Ex 8:7).

13. He caused the frogs to die (Ex 8:8-15).

14. He converted the dust to lice: third plague (Ex 8:16-19; the magicians could not do this, Ex 8:18-

15. He created flies: fourth plague (Ex 8:20-24).

16. He made Goshen exempt from flies (Ex 8:22).

17. He removed the flies from Egypt (Ex 8:29-32).

18. The murrain disease was imposed on Egyptian stock: fifth plague (Ex 9:1-7).

19. The stock of Israel was exempt (Ex 9:4-7).

20. He made boils from ashes: sixth plague (Ex 9:8-12).

21. Hail and fire came: seventh plague (Ex 9:13-35).

22. Goshen was exempt from the hail and fire (Ex 9:26).

23. Moses stopped the hail and fire (Ex 9:28-35).

24. Locusts descended: eighth plague (Ex 10:1-15)

25. The locusts were removed (Ex 10:16-20).

26. Darkness came: ninth plague (Ex 10:21-29).

27. Goshen was exempt from the total darkness (Ex 10:23).

28. Death came to Egypt's firstborn: tenth plague (Ex 11-12).

29. Israel's firstborn were exempt from death (Ex 11:7-10).

30. Moses made a path through the Red Sea, congealing the water (Ex 14:21-22).

31. He melted the ice of Red Sea (Ex 14:26-28).

32. The healing waters of Marah (Ex 15:23-26).

33. Bread from heaven (Ex 16:4-35; Num 11).

34. Quail to eat (Ex 16:8-13).

35. Water from the rock (Ex 17:1-7).

36. His victory over Midian (Ex 17:11-13).

37. He quenched the fire of death (Num 11:2).

38. The healing of Miriam (Num 12:13-16).

39. The earth swallowed the rebels (Num 16:28-33).

40. Moses stopped the plague (Num 16:44-50).

41. Water from the rock (Num 20:10-13).

42. The healing of Israel (Num 21:5-9; John 3:14).

Sixteen other miracles that God performed when Moses was present (Ex 7:10)

1. God's glory filling tabernacle (Ex 40:34).

2. Fire consuming sacrifices (Lev 9:24).

3. Fire killing priests (Lev 10:2).

4. The Fire which consumed some people (Num 11:2).

5. The fire was quenched (Num 11:2).

6. A month's supply of quails for about 6,000,000 people (Num 11:19-35).

7. The leprosy that was fixed upon Miriam (Num 12:10).

8. The healing of Miriam (Num 12:13-16).

9. The plague upon ten spies (Num 14:37).

10. The earth swallowed the rebels (Num 16:32).

11. The fire which consumed some people (Num 16:35).

12. The plague which killed 14,700 people (Num 16:49).

13. Aaron's rod that bore almonds (Num 17:8).

14. Water from the rock (Num 20:11).

15. The healing of Israel (Num 21:5-9).

16. The plague which killed 24,000 people (Num 25:9).

(from Dake Annotated Reference Bible © 2007 by Dake Publishing. All rights reserved in U.S.A. and Other Countries.)

(Dake Annotated Reference Bible, n.d.)

Bibliography

Blue Letter Bible. (n.d.). *Strong's G169 - akathartos.*
Retrieved from blueletterbible.org:
https://www.blueletterbible.org/lexicon/g169/kjv/tr
/0-1/

Blue Letter Bible. (n.d.). *Strong's G2896 - krazō.* Retrieved
from blueletterbible.org:
https://www.blueletterbible.org/lexicon/g2896/kjv/t
r/0-1/

Blue Letter Bible. (n.d.). *Strong's G4151 - pneuma.* Retrieved
from blueletterbible.org:
https://www.blueletterbible.org/lexicon/g4151/kjv/t
r/0-1/

Blue Letter Bible. (n.d.). *Strong's G4682 - sparassō.* Retrieved
from blueletterbible.org:
https://www.blueletterbible.org/lexicon/g4682/kjv/t
r/0-1/

Blue Letter Bible. (n.d.). *Strong's G4828 - symmartyreō.*
Retrieved from blueletterbible.org:
https://www.blueletterbible.org/lexicon/g4828/kjv/t
r/0-1/

Blue Letter Bible. (n.d.). *Strong's G5319 - phaneroō.*
Retrieved from blueletterbible.org:
https://www.blueletterbible.org/lexicon/g5319/kjv/t
r/0-1/

Blue Letter Bible. (n.d.). *Strong's H7462 - rā ā*. Retrieved from Blue Letter Bible: https://www.blueletterbible.org/lexicon/h7462/kjv/wlc/0-1/

Blue Letter Bilble. (n.d.). *Strong's G2347 - thlipsis*. Retrieved from blueletterbible.org: https://www.blueletterbible.org/lexicon/g2347/esv/mgnt/0-1/

Dake Annotated Reference Bible. (n.d.). *42-Miracles-and-wonders-done-through-Moses*. Retrieved from faithfamilybillings.com: https://faithfamilybillings.com/wp-content/uploads/2016/08/42-Miracles-and-wonders-done-through-Moses.pdf

Got Questions. (n.d.). *Is epilepsy mentioned in the Bible?* Retrieved from gotquestions.org: https://www.gotquestions.org/epilepsy-Bible.html

Got Questions. (n.d.). *Who was Smith Wigglesworth?* Retrieved from goquestions.org: https://www.gotquestions.org/Smith-Wigglesworth.html

Healing and Revival.com. (n.d.). *Apostle of Faith*. Retrieved from healingandrevival.com: https://healingandrevival.com/BioSWigglesworth.htm

Healing and Revival.com. (n.d.). *Healing and Mass Evangelism*. Retrieved from healingandrevival.com: https://healingandrevival.com/BioTLOsborn.htm

Healing and Revival.com. (n.d.). *I Believe in Miracles*. Retrieved from healingandrevival.com: https://healingandrevival.com/BioKKuhlman.htm

Healing and Revival.com. (n.d.). *The Miracle Man*. Retrieved from healingandrevival.com: https://healingandrevival.com/BioAAAllen.htm

Isgrigg, D. D. (2021, Mar 24). *Who is Oral Roberts?* Retrieved from danieldisgrigg.com: https://danieldisgrigg.com/2021/03/24/who-is-oral-roberts/

Publishing, N. L. (n.d.). *William Branham – The Prophet of Controversy*. Retrieved from newlifepublishing.co.uk: https://www.newlifepublishing.co.uk/articles/faith/william-branham-the-prophet-of-controversy/

Shilling, E. (2016, Oct 13). *The Unverifiable Legend of the Early 20th-Century Preacher Who Raised 14 People from the Dead*. Retrieved from atlasobscura.com: https://www.atlasobscura.com/articles/the-unverifiable-legend-of-the-early-20thcentury-preacher-who-raised-14-people-from-the-dead

Society, P. o. (n.d.). *http://www.scielo.org.za/*. Retrieved from On-line version ISSN 2305-0853: http://www.scielo.org.za/scielo.php?script=sci_arttext&pid=S2305-

08532014000200004#:~:text=The%20leper%20in%2
0the%20story,warn%20people%20of%20their%20illn
ess

Other Books By the Author:

Amazon
https://rebrand.ly/Ivan-Thompson-Amazon

Audible
https://rebrand.ly/Ivan-Thompson-Audible

Here is a list of the e-book & print titles that I have available on Amazon:

- *25 Essential Bible Verses for Christian Business Leaders
- 25 Versículos Esenciales de la Biblia Para Líderes de Negocios Cristianos
- *25 Bible Verses for Dads
- 25 Versículos Bíblicos para Papás: Un Diario de Reflexión
- *A Tsunami of Sadness
- Un Tsunami de Tristeza
- *Hope Deferred Overcoming Discouragement and Faltering Hope
- Esperanza Frustrada: Superando el Desánimo y la Falta de Esperanza
- Finding Next A Book of Divine Seasons
- Financial Testimonies Stories of God's Grace and Provision
- Financial Testimonies II

- *First Responders a Revelation of the Love of Jesus
- Primeros en Responder: "Una Revelación del Amor de Jesús" (Spanish Edition)
- Increasing Your Skills and Abilities in Any Area
- Letters to Build a Young Man's Confidence
- *Lifesaving The Importance of Hearing the Voice of God
- PODRÍA SALVAR TU VIDA: La importancia de escuchar la voz de Dios
- *Lifesaving Volume II Hardening Your Heart to the Voice of God
- Podría Salvar Tu Vida Volumen II : Endurecer el Corazón a la Voz de Dios
- *The Bible Promises of Healing 16 Letters for Mom
- Promesas de Curación de la Biblia : 16 Cartas para Mamá
- The Making of a Great America Where the Founding Fathers and the Church Fell Short
- The Making of a Great America Uprooting the Spirit of Racism
- The Making of a Great America Made in the Image of Trump
- *You Should Detours and Distractions to Divine Destiny
- Usted Debería: Distracciones Y Desvíos Del Destino Divino
- Fit @ 50

- <u>No Grandma It's an e-book</u>
- <u>The Air Force's Black Ceiling</u>
- <u>The Air Force's Black Pilot Training Experience</u>
- <u>The Air Force's Black Pilot State of the Union</u>

***Also available in Spanish**

Here is a list of the audiobook titles that I have available on Audible:

- **The Making of a Great America: Where the Founding Fathers and the Church Fell Short**
- **The Making of a Great America: Made in Trump's Image**
- **A Tsunami of Sadness**
- **Financial Testimonies: Stories of God's Favor, Grace, and Provision**
- **25 Essential Bible Verses for Christian Business Leaders**
- **25 Versículos Esenciales de la Biblia para Líderes de Negocios Cristianos**
- **You Should Distractions & Detours to Divine Destiny**
- **Usted Debería: Distracciones Y Desvíos Del Destino Divino**
- **The Bible Promises of Healing 16 Letters for Mom**
- **First Responders a Revelation of the Love of Jesus**

- **25 Essential Bible Verses for Dads**
- **Increasing Your Skills and Abilities in Any Area**
- **Letters to Build a Young Man's Confidence**
- **No Grandma It's an e-Book!**
- **The Air Force's Black Ceiling**

www.ingramcontent.com/pod-product-compliance
Lightning Source LLC
Chambersburg PA
CBHW050808260726
48660CB00004B/1317